# WARRIOR NURSE
## PTSD AND HEALING

Sarah L. Blum

Black Rose Writing | Texas

©2025 by Sarah L. Blum
All rights reserved. No part of this book may be reproduced, stored in a retrieval system or transmitted in any form or by any means without the prior written permission of the publishers, except by a reviewer who may quote brief passages in a review to be printed in a newspaper, magazine or journal.

The author grants the final approval for this literary material.

First printing

Some names and identifying details may have been changed to protect the privacy of individuals.

ISBN: 978-1-68513-569-0
PUBLISHED BY BLACK ROSE WRITING
www.blackrosewriting.com

Printed in the United States of America
Suggested Retail Price (SRP) $21.95

*Warrior Nurse* is printed in Minion Pro

\*As a planet-friendly publisher, Black Rose Writing does its best to eliminate unnecessary waste to reduce paper usage and energy costs, while never compromising the reading experience. As a result, the final word count vs. page count may not meet common expectations.

# Praise for
# WARRIOR NURSE

"Some people still believe that no American women served in Vietnam during that war. They are wrong. Sarah Blum describes in graphic and shocking detail her experiences as an Army operating room nurse at the 12$^{th}$ Evacuation Hospital in Cu Chi, reputed to be the busiest combat hospital in Vietnam in 1967. She shares the life-shattering experiences that drove her down into the madness of PTSD. I well recall when she ran through the hospital screaming, "Kill! Kill, Kill!" Neither she nor her colleagues understood what was happening to her at that time. When she returned home, she devoted her life to seeking answers. She offers a wealth of information in this book, as well as myriad resources to help PTSD sufferers deal with their anguish and move on with their lives."
**–Dr. Beth Parks, former Army operating room nurse, 7th Surgical Hospital (MASH) and 12$^{th}$ Evacuation Hospital, Cu Chi, Vietnam, 1966-67**

"From the opening of *Warrior Nurse* where the author reveals she served at the 12th Evac Hospital in Cu Chi, Vietnam, she had me. I served at the same location for a year of that insane Vietnam war. I could immediately identify. Likewise, with much of the remainder of this superbly-written *cri de coeur*, though I haven't Nurse Blum's medical expertise. More than forty years later as a retired Army colonel, I sat in the lobby of the main building at the National Military Medical Center and talked with a USAF triple amputee who was a tragic casualty of yet another insane war. Today, I now know viscerally what suicide, post-traumatic stress, and deeply-felt and haunting feelings of guilt have done to tens of thousands of veterans. Every single American citizen should be compelled to read this book to gain stunning insight into what we have done to these young men and women since the first one of them set foot in Vietnam, followed by hundreds of thousands more in Iraq, Afghanistan, Somalia, Syria, Ukraine, and Gaza. And most should weep for their neglect. Then, do something about it."
**–Lawrence Wilkerson, Col, USA (Ret) and former chief of staff to the U.S. Secretary of State**

"*Warrior Nurse: PTSD and Healing* by Sarah L. Blum is a much needed and informative read written from the heart of a true hero. Blum has done amazing work as a U.S. Army OR Nurse during the Vietnam War, nurse psychotherapist to emotionally wounded veterans, and now as an author. As a military daughter & survivor of suicide loss, this book has given me a deeper understanding into the illness of PTSD and the mental wounds that my father, and other soldiers and military support personnel, returned home with. If more veterans are able to heal their PTSD with the treatment modalities Blum recommends, we will be able to reduce rates of soldier suicide and improve the quality of life for those who served. Warrior Nurse is an asset to those looking to heal their PTSD & move forward from their trauma, and to military family members who are seeking help and supporting their wounded warriors."

–**Amily D'Nas, author of the award- winning novel** *Beneath the Swaying Willow*

"In *Warrior Nurse, PTSD and Healing*, Sarah Blum takes us along on an emotional roller coaster journey that begins with her patriotic yearning to serve her country, winds us through the depths of despair in her time as an operating nurse on the jungle battlefields of Vietnam during the height of the war, and then submerges us in the seemingly relentless quicksand of PTSD. But it's not just a story from afar about this horrid invisible wound so many of our soldiers bring back home with them, rather, it's a tale of her own personal sufferings that begin with her encounter with "Johnny," and how she not only learned what this strange ailment was and how to deal with it, but more so, how she became an agent of hope, helping others to find light where there was none. And it's "Johnny," in a more spiritual sort of way, that helps her become a helper.

*Warrior Nurse, PTSD and Healing* is a story of the realities and horrors of war, and how so many are left with the scars deep inside that require more than just antibiotics and a gauze wrap. She shows how it's understanding and therapy that can be used as the IV drip to help make the pain dull, maybe even make life worth living once again. In a well written "diary" of sorts, Sarah takes us from her time as a patient – mired in the lava pits of PTSD at its worst – to a healer, helping others that have fallen into that same burning hole.

So, in essence, it's really a story of hope. Something we can all use these days.

A wonderful and powerful read."

–**Jim Bartlett, author of more than a hundred short stories, including** *The Grand Adventure*, **winner of the Spillwords Press' best publication for April 2024**

"It took me several years to realize that I did not leave those memories behind in Vietnam, they were buried deep in my brain and slowly began to emerge with dreams, sights and sounds. It took me years with counseling from many different counselors to get a grasp of how the Vietnam war affected me.

Sarah has researched PTSD and explains everything in detail and I wish that had this book when I was going through my difficult time. I believe that counselors who are seeing Veterans, especially Vietnam Veterans, need this book in their library. I also think that Vietnam veterans who are still experiencing the aftermath of the Vietnam war, need to be given the opportunity to read this book.

My congratulations to Sarah for her tenacity to stay on task and complete this important book which I believe will help many who suffer from PTSD."
**–Connie Evans, Ret. CMDR, USPHS Corps, Fmr, CPT US Army Nurse Corps 12th Evacuation Hospital staff CuChi, Republic of S. Vietnam**

"Beginning with her experiences of the horrid realities of war as an OR nurse in Vietnam, Sarah Blum describes her lifelong healing journey toward finding healing modalities and hope, which she shares with the reader. She poses questions we all ought to be asking about war.

Blum served soldiers by mending their mangled bodies while she lived in constant fear at the hectic evacuation hospital amid the worst fighting, in Cu Chi. She describes the everyday tasks, routines, sounds, smells, and dangers of her life as an OR nurse in raw, vivid stories. From bombings and attacks to the intimate proximity of Viet Cong tunnel entrances next to outhouses, danger and fear of death or injury stalked every moment. The perils coming from these tunnels undermining Cu Chi became so infamous that they are now a tourist attraction.

Blum's stories give authenticity to the wisdom gained through her lifelong journey of restoring health and function to her "shell-shocked" body, mind, and soul, followed by decades of guiding others in their healing from PTSD. She now gifts her wisdom to others in this book. Blum offers a host of complementary healing modalities and encourages "victims" to become "cocreators" of their own destiny, knowing that their lives will be enhanced by healing."
**–Linda Jean Shepherd, author of *Lifting the Veil: The Feminine Face of Science***

"Post-traumatic stress is a very reasonable response to very unreasonable circumstances. Faced with too-common horrors from warfare to sexual assault, it is understandable that individuals develop defenses to manage the pain, shame and residual fear borne of these memories. These coping mechanisms only becoming problematic when they hinder the ability to fully engage in life mindfully.

Decorated Vietnam veteran Sarah Blum has seen it all, from the front lines to the homefront and she's spent decades experimenting with myriad methods and mindsets to undo the damage done to her soul. Her superpower is bringing order to chaos, whether it be imbuing compassion within the care of soldiers in a Vietnam MASH unit or spelling out systemic change to care for contemporary victims of MST.

Post-traumatic stress is an epidemic; *Warrior Nurse: PTSD and Healing* prescribes the cure."

**–Warren Etheredge, Founder, The Red Badge Project (http://theredbadgeproject.org) Founder, The Warren Report**

"Sarah Blum brings it. She opens her heart and gives you a rare and vivid glimpse into the life of a veteran and caregiver, and then offers fantastic help for those people suffering with or trying to understand PTSD. She's come through that struggle herself, and so speaks with both authority and expertise. This book is for anyone who has known the ravages of war or who loves someone who has. It's a gift."

**–William Kenower, author of *Everyone Has What It Takes: A Writer's Guide to the End of Self-Doubt***

"*Warrior Nurse: PTSD and Healing* is an invaluable guide for veterans. But it's also an intelligent and heartfelt memoir that all readers will find compelling. Blum's vivid evocation of her year in Viet Nam and its aftermath are unforgettable. Reading this book has changed me."

**–Barbara Turner-Vesselago, author of *Writing Without a Parachute: The Art of Freefall* and *Freefall Into Fiction: Finding Form (Hachette).***

"*Warrior Nurse: PTSD and Healing* documents Sarah Blum's story of becoming an Army nurse who began her "world tour" in Vietnam in 1967 with the war raging.

The narrative starts in media res six months into Sarah's tour of duty. As she steps into the operating room of the 12th Evacuation Hospital in Cu Chi, the busiest and most dangerous hospital in Vietnam's Iron Triangle, Sarah encounters Johnny, a young soldier whose entire lower body has been shattered by a 105-mm artillery shell.

From this moment of shock, horror, and penetrating sadness to the completion of this book, some 58 years later, we walk with Sarah as she learns to heal through comradeship, writing, and a desire to understand her brain and body. The physical, emotional, and spiritual journeys she chronicles offer valuable insight for all service members who struggle with returning home, their families, and the general public. The resources available in chapters such as Chapter 11, "Support and Adjunct to Therapy," could help others "reclaim" parts of themselves and cope with their trauma.

Blum's second book is not only a personal story; it also documents and preserves women's contributions to the military and provides insights that could inform policy changes."

**–James M. Dubinsky, LTC, US Army (ret.) teaches at Virginia Tech, where he has helped begin an initiative focusing on veterans and their families (Veterans in Society/Veterans Studies).**

# Acknowledgements

This book would not be a reality without the genuine support from my many veteran friends in our Council of Return especially, Ryan Mielcarek, Crystal Dandridge, Danny Medoff, Jessica Talley, and my writing teacher, Warren Etheredge, in the Red Badge Veterans Writing Class. I also acknowledge the listening ear of my veteran friend, Elizabeth Bissett, the many adventures we had and the things she taught me about service dogs.

My daughter Lorna Pella has been a long-time supporter for much that I have done and continue to do. Her constant love and support mean the world to me and have helped me continue with what I am called to do. My son-in-law Mark Pella has helped me with so many things in my home and my life that made it possible for me to write. My writing group helped me learn so much about writing and to have the confidence to write what is in my heart and I am grateful for each of them: Bruce Taylor aka Mr. Magic Realism, Roberta Gregory, Jim Bartlett, and Linda Shepherd. All great fiction writers and Art Gomez, an amazing poet.

I would still be stuck in the throes of my PTSD without Elaine Childs-Gowell, who was my therapist from 1981-1987; who taught me how to heal myself and others and to use my passion for that purpose and so much more. I am truly grateful for her and all that she taught me. She remains in my heart even though she left this world years ago.

Without the work and dedication of Bessel Van Der Kolk, I would not have understood PTSD or the many ways to work with it to bring about healing. I attended many of his seminars over the years and have read and reread his book: *The Body Keeps the Score*. All veterans owe gratitude to Dr. Van Der Kolk for his ground- breaking work in healing PTSD.

Gratitude goes out to all the soldiers I have met over the years who have stood with me and supported me in my efforts to heal myself and others, including those who came through the operating room at the 12th Evacuation Hospital during 1967, causing me to face challenges that both hurt deeply and led to my healing. I especially acknowledge Jim Vines who was part of the Manchus and who I was fortunate to meet in person years after his injuries from October 1967. Jim brought me to Texas in June 2014, to the Vietnam Memorial there, where I met many of the other Manchus. My heart is still there with all of you. Deep gratitude for Jim and all his buddies. We miss you, Jim. Here is a picture of Jim when he met me at the airport. You can see his hand on my left shoulder.

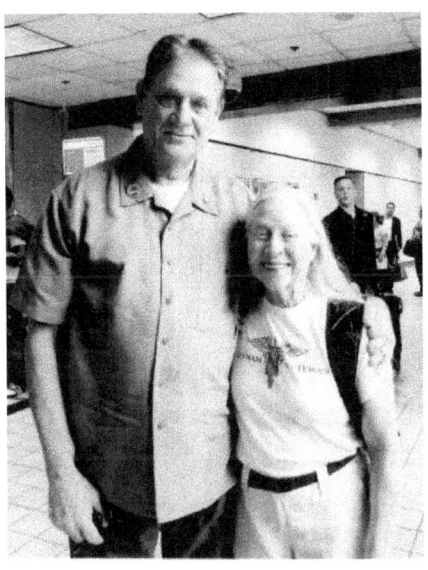

1. Picture of Jim Vines meeting me at the airport in Dallas, Texas June 2014. Photo from private phone.

# Foreword

Since its establishment on February 2, 1901, the Army Nurse Corps has cared for soldiers during peace and war. In World War II, they deployed to the European Theater before fighting soldiers because they were needed. In the 124 years that nurses have provided care to the troops, they have always volunteered for that duty. We are most proud of our support to the troops and their families, because we were there because we desired to be.

There are many books written about the Vietnam era and the Vietnam War. Many of the accounts are conflicting about why we were there, why we stayed for a lengthy period and whether our participation in the conflict would justify the 50,000 casualties recorded. There were many, many demonstrations in cities, towns and college campuses all over the United States. Many young men left the country to avoid the draft or to escape enlistment. It is the only war or conflict in which U. S. troops participated and did not receive a hero's welcome when they returned to American soil. It was a time of great turmoil in our Nation.

Sarah Blum, the author of *Warrior Nurse: PTSD & Healing*, was a nurse who decided that she should join the Army and go to Vietnam, because that was where she was needed. Approximately 7,500 women served in Vietnam and the majority were nurses. The first half of the book is all about her Vietnam experiences. She was a keen observer, both on and off duty, and she writes about her observations in exquisite detail. The hospital to which she was assigned was so close to the battlefield she could hear the helicopters before they arrived with casualties. The writer gives such vivid accounts of her work experiences in the operating room until the reader may imagine that she/he was there with her. Despite all the tragedies and sufferings of war, the military was able to teach the health care community of the world how to use helicopters for rapid transport of the wounded and sick.

The second half of Sarah's book is her own treatment for PTSD or post traumatic stress disorder. The author must take great pride in her willingness to reveal much intimate and personal information to readers. It reflects the great confidence she has in herself after having survived wartime experiences and its aftermath, recovered from PTSD, became a nurse psycho- therapist and dedicated herself to helping others. She is a living example of a nurse who cares about herself and others.

*Nurse Warrior: PTSD & Healing* should be read because it is a story about all aspects of war from a nurse who was there and paying attention. It is commendable that she took the time to make astute observations, took the time to make assessments and to work through them. In this memoir, we have benefit of the demonstrated courage and caring of an Army nurse who served valiantly in defense of the Nation.

**Clara L. Adams-Ender, RN, BSN, MSN, MMAS, FAAN, CNAA, LLAN, PhD (hon)**
**Brigadier General, U.S.Army, Retired**


In November of 1965 after completing a five -year surgical residency I was drafted and sent to Vietnam as the Chief of Surgery for the 12th evacuation Hospital. Sarah Blum volunteered to go to Vietnam and she became my scrub nurse. Many non- medical people believe that a scrub nurse just hands off instruments, but that job is so much more. A scrub nurse must gather and pack the right instruments and have them ready to go when the surgeon reaches out his hand. A critically wounded patient bleeding to death on the operating table is not the time to search for the right instruments. A good scrub nurse must anticipate the surgeons every move and need as the case proceeds, and when the hand reaches out the nurse delivers the proper clamp or suture without even asking. Sarah Blum was marvelous and her abilities saved many lives, but her talents didn't end when the operations were over.

Most of us shut out the horrors by moving on to the next patient but not Sarah. She carried her compassion with her. What were these wounded going to think when they awoke with paralysis and amputations.? How were they going to cope, how were they going to heal the deep phycological wounds that wars produce and what could she do to help. Those were the questions Sarah carried with her for the rest of her life.

Still in the army when she returned from Vietnam, she asked to be assigned to the orthopedic ward at Madigan Army Hospital. Listening, encouraging and counseling these mutilated young men must have been the hardest job a nurse could request, but Sarah chose it and began to learn about PTSD , a disease that hadn't even been named yet and wasn't officially added to the American Psychiatric Association's manual until 1980 .

This book is Sarah's inspiring story. The story of a brave compassionate woman who made a difference . For any who want to learn about the tremendous contributions nurses made in both the line of battle in Vietnam and in fighting the psychological ravages of war participants carry with them, this book is an inspiring read.

**Stuart M. Poticha MD, FACS**
**Chief of surgery, 12th Evacuation Hospital**
**CuChi, Vietnam**
**Emeritus Associate Professor of Surgery Northwestern University Medical School**

# WARRIOR NURSE

# Table of Contents

**Acknowledgements**

**Introduction**

| | | |
|---|---|---|
| **Chapter 1** | Standing in their Blood | 1 |
| **Chapter 2** | Up Close and Personal in Vietnam – Part 1 | 17 |
| **Chapter 3** | Up Close and Personal in Vietnam – Part 2 | 44 |
| **Chapter 4** | Home from the War | 68 |
| **Chapter 5** | The Effects of my Vietnam Experiences | 83 |
| **Chapter 6** | The Healing Begins | 96 |
| **Chapter 7** | PTSD and Healing | 115 |
| **Chapter 8** | Understanding PTSD | 124 |
| **Chapter 9** | Our Body, Brain and PTSD | 135 |
| **Chapter 10** | Essentials of Treatment | 144 |
| **Chapter 11** | Support and Adjuncts to Therapy | 170 |
| **Chapter 12** | Attitudes and Beliefs | 219 |

**References** 230

**Appendix:** 231
- Group Therapy Contract — 231
- Think Structure — 236
- Phantasy Check Out — 237
- Client Rights — 237
- Clearing Structure — 238
- Types of Work — 240
- EFT (Emotional Freedom Technique) — 241
- My Letters to Dad — 244

# Introduction

In 2006, I felt called to write about women who had served in the military. I believed that like me, they all had their own stories to tell. I was willing to put my own time, energy and money into listening to their stories and compiling them into a book.

I was two years into the project when I met an author at a women's drum circle. We met in the kitchen around the potluck food. Her name is Linda Shepherd and her book is: *Lifting the Veil: The Feminine Face of Science*. She talked with me about writing, the Pacific Northwest Writers Association, their annual conference and being part of a writers' group. I told her I would love to be part of the writers' group, and within weeks, I attended my first group to meet the other authors and respond to their questions about me. I found out that the group had been in existence for better than ten years and was made up of talented authors who were published in quite a variety of genres. I felt honored to be asked to join them since I was such a novice. I also followed Linda's suggestion to learn more about the PNWA Writers conference. When I called the association number, I was fortunate in that I was able to speak directly to the president, Pam Binder. She was delightful, informative, and supportive. She told me about the upcoming conference in July that I had already missed the early bird deadline for, but since I only just learned about it, she gave me the early bird price. In addition, she explained how to write a proposal and encouraged me to do that. She suggested I bring copies with me so that I could get appointments with agents and editors and have my proposals ready. She also told me how to write a pitch and to have that prepared as well. It was both overwhelming and exciting to be entering this whole new world.

I became a member of the writers' group and started learning a lot right away. I felt supported by these seasoned writers and I contributed my own perspective to their writing. I also attended the writers' conference where the energy was amazingly electric. I took many notes, learned for three days, met wonderful people, had fun, and met with agents and editors. The biggest surprise was going to a drum circle that Saturday night instead of to the Saturday conference event and then returning home to a message from two of the agents. The message said basically they read through my proposal, were impressed and were offering me a contract. Wow!

That was the beginning of being part of the world of authors, agents, and publishing. The next year, I went to the conference again and that time I learned about the relationship between author and agent and realized that what I was experiencing with my agents was not helpful. Doubts came up regularly with what seemed to be complex and unhealthy communications from the agents. The workshop confirmed it. Even though it was a bit scary to fire my agents so quickly, I believed it was for the best and felt very relieved. I did not want to stay connected to people who did not communicate clearly, since that clarity would be essential to me.

After another year went by, learning so much more, I decided to turn over what I had written to someone who could give me feedback. I was overwhelmed with the amount of feedback I received, the quality and content of it. It took me three months to absorb it all and take it to heart. Doing that required that I completely shift the focus of the book from women veterans to the sexual assault of women in the military. There had been several stories of women who were sexually assaulted while serving. The editor pointed those out and said the direction I was going would not result in publication but if I narrowed the focus, it would more likely be picked up for publication. Changing the focus like that required that I contact the women I had already received stories from and let them know of the change. Many of the women did not want to be part of the new focus and their stories would not have fit anyway. Making the change also meant I had to eliminate my own detailed story of service and the impact it had.

I shifted all of my story to a different file and put it away. Later, much later, more like 2014, my story became the basis for this book. It was difficult for me to get back into it and focus on writing about my own PTSD and healing process, as well as write about what PTSD is and address how to heal it. Over the years I struggled to write as I would lose interest and motivation, and even at times, lose faith in myself that I could write it. During that period, I was engulfed in the callings of my profession as a nurse psychotherapist and my personal life. It wasn't until 2020 when I met Ryan Mielcarek and was introduced to Veteran Rites, Path with Art and the Red Badge Writing Class, that I felt enough support and motivation to get back to writing the book.

Being part of the Council of Return (circles of initiates who did ceremony within Veteran Rites) with so many wonderful veterans was key to my being able to complete this book. I had a safe place to go every week online to share my feelings and things that were coming up in my writing or in general. The other veterans listened and I felt their support. I did the same for them, listened and supported them. That continues to this day. I also attended the Red Badge Writing Class weekly and again had support for my writing among all of us veterans. Sometime in the last year I also had the good fortune to be part of a women's healing room with women veterans online (Red Feather Ranch) one day a week. Between all those support groups, I had no excuse not to complete the book. As I write this, I am pages away from completion and feeling great. I sincerely hope that what I have written will serve each and every person who reads it in helpful ways.

My intention, as I write this book, is not only to help provide some understanding about what PTSD is to the reader, but how to better deal with its effects, and even help to heal it. There will be some complicated professional language included at times, but be assured that I will break it down and explain it so it is clear and relatable to you.

# Chapter 1
# STANDING IN THEIR BLOOD

I had been an army operating room nurse at the 12th Evacuation Hospital Cu Chi, Vietnam for about six months when Johnny was brought in. Three of our surgeons were alerted and showed up for him. Johnny was nineteen years old with red hair, bright blue eyes and a strong healthy body — but all of that was obscured by the severity of his injuries. Johnny had been hit by American artillery, a 105 mm Howitzer to be exact. He was brought to us by dust-off helicopter within minutes of being blasted. His legs were barely hanging on by skin and muscle; the bones of his legs were shattered; his penis testicles and buttocks were full of shrapnel; and his thighs, lower legs, and buttocks were black, ugly, blasted open, mutilated and bloody. He was losing a lot of blood and he had clamps on his major arteries in the groin to keep him from bleeding out before we could do surgery.

Because our team had been at the 12th Evac for between four-six months, we were well trained and honed by our experiences up until that moment. We all looked at Johnny and no one was sure what we could do for him. I was scrubbed in and ready professionally, but emotionally horrified by what I was seeing. An all-too-common experience. *Would he want to live with only half a body? How would his body function after this? Could we just let him die? What if he didn't die? What can we fix?* I could feel something like lead in my stomach, my own body was tense and I was holding my breath. I looked at Dr. Henry, our urologist, and saw his eyes full of water while pleading not to have to do this, his jaw tightly clenched as he said, "How do we decide what to do? When will this fucking destruction of human life end!?" He was making fists with his gloved hands as he said it. I felt a welling up of the fiery energy of anger, rage and passion that I had come to live with for the past six months. I could see Dr. Travis' face contort with his well-held feelings. He was our orthopedic surgeon, and Dr. Dynan, our general surgeon, was shaking his head.

It seemed like those long surreal moments, of seeing the underside of Johnny's bloodied and blasted legs, penis, scrotum and buttocks, were held together in suspended animation. We could hear the anesthesia machine with its loud simulated rhythmic respiratory sounds keeping Johnny's lungs working, yet we were barely breathing. None of the three doctors wanted to make the decision.

Dr. Henry and I were with Johnny for four hours standing in his blood as it ran down the sheets onto the floor, onto us, and our shoes. Dr. Travis and Dynan were able to leave earlier after their part was done. Dr. Travis and I took off Johnny's useless legs, while Dr. Henry had to repair his testicles, his penis, and urethra. Johnny ended up with big skin flaps loosely covering over the inside of his pelvis and hips when we sent him to post-op. He went from having a whole healthy body to having only half of a badly blasted and mangled body. Now, his body went from his head to his pelvis and there was nothing beyond that, so there was nowhere to attach artificial legs. It was a devastating loss that I could feel in my own body with a heaviness in my chest, a lead like lump in my stomach and an overwhelming sense of despair.

I started that day wondering: *How does any human being do this to another? How can I keep doing this? How can I see any more young men with their bodies and lives destroyed— and for what? Why are we here? Why are we doing this?*

I heard their screams in my head. I saw their faces in my mind's eye and what I couldn't forget were their pleading eyes and the smell of their blood. I had been feeling exhausted when Johnny showed me the worst of the horrors in war, and if I had not already been emotionally numb to it, I don't know if I could have gone on. I wondered if Johnny would survive or if he would even want to live the way he would end up.

That night when I was off duty and finally able to take a shower, I could not get the smell of Johnny's blood out of my head and nose. No matter how many cold showers I took or how much soap I used, the smell of his blood would not go away. One of the worst things for me about working in surgery was that I always had a lot of blood all over me and would be standing in it for hours. Sometimes I felt like I couldn't get it off my skin or the metallic smell out of my head: fresh and old blood, in my nose and in my head— their blood, my brothers' blood, Johnny's blood. Even when it was washed off and I knew it was gone, I could still smell it. After taking that cold shower (because we did not have hot water), I was wide-awake and needed to talk. That night my whole body felt like it was made of the heaviest metal and my legs could only drag rather than walk. I wanted to cry forever, yet could not shed even one tear because all my emotions were locked up tight. The other nurses in the hooch (long wooden structure with individual personal spaces divided by bamboo netting) were laughing and listening to music, but I could not join in this time. I could not make the shift. I managed to drag my now clean body, filled with the smell of my brother's blood, over to the olive drab army phone. I turned the crank several times and waited for the familiar sound of the Aussie operator voice after I asked, "Are you working?"

I had been reaching out to the Aussies for months when I needed human contact apart from the war. There were a bunch of Aussie soldiers who ran the communications system in Vietnam, which included the phones. Finally, I heard the voice I was waiting for "working," said the familiar sounding Aussie voice. Many of the Aussies were from Sydney so I often called them by that name.

"Hi, Sydney, this is Sarah. Can you take a few minutes to talk with me?"

"Yes, I can do that. Did you have a bad experience?"

"More than my emotions can handle right now." I told him about Johnny's wounds and that I couldn't get the smell of his blood or the memory of his wounds out of my head. "Can you talk to me for a while and tell me about Australia, where you live and what it's like there?" My conversations lasted only about ten to fifteen minutes but were comforting to me. They took my mind off of the horrors I dealt with and pain I felt from that war.

Three days later, I entered the operating room (OR) and saw that I was the first one there. I came in through the door closest to the wards and hooches. At the opposite end was a door that led to our outhouse and the tunnel opening that the Viet Cong used. That tunnel opening was about six feet from the outhouse door. The war raged all around us including in those tunnels underneath our hospital. As I walked forward, I could see that in front of the door at the other end of the OR, was a stretcher… and on it was a big bump… covered by a sheet. As I walked toward the stretcher, I saw the foot-end of it covered with a white sheet that laid flat on the bed. I continued to see the flat, flat, flat as my eyes followed up to the middle of the stretcher where the bump started. I continued to walk slowly toward the heap — and then I saw him. Emerging from that hump was the head of a young, red headed blue-eyed guy about nineteen years old. *Oh no, it's Johnny!* At that moment when I saw his face, something in me cracked. I was on my way to say something to him, I don't know what, but I couldn't do it. *What could I say?*

I felt all the emotions from the previous six months come up inside me all at once: the intense pressure of anger, outrage, deep grief, and utter helplessness. Then I felt something snap inside me; I ran past Johnny and out the door. I continued running around the hospital, all the way around with my fist in the air, crazed and enraged shouting and screaming at the helicopters overhead, "KILL! KILL! KILL! THAT IS ALL YOU KNOW HOW TO DO. STOP THE KILLING! NO MORE DESTRUCTION!" The next thing I remember is standing in front of my chief nurse's desk telling her, "I can't take it anymore! You've gotta get me out of the OR! Put me on the malaria ward or something!" And she said, in typical army fashion for Vietnam, "You'll be OK, you just need a rest." That was the psychiatric protocol for the Vietnam conflict— deny any psychological effects of the war on those serving and tell them they just needed a rest or a break and they will be OK.[1]

She sent me to the in-country rest and recovery center (R and R) located in Vung Tau. I was able to leave the next day to go there. As the helicopter flew near Vung Tau, I could see the beautiful beach, the South China Sea and a big green hill. A little further on, the helicopter turned around that hill and into view came army vehicles, a beach area filled with jeeps, trucks, Army Personnel Carriers (APC's) and other army equipment. It was an ugly contrast of olive drab (OD) green everywhere and the loveliness of the beach obscured by it. In fact, the sand itself, seemed to be OD green and brown in that area.

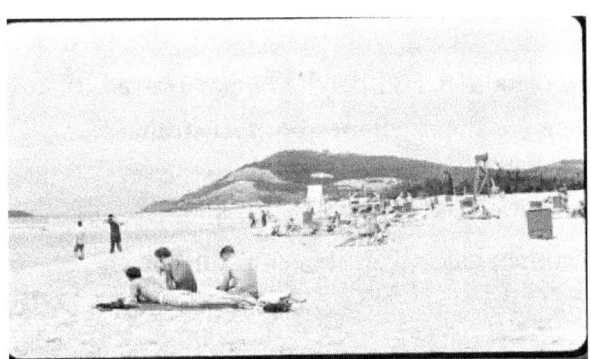

2. Beach at Vung Tau where I was sent for three days in March 1967. Photo is a slide from my Pentax camera.

As soon as I could, I headed to the Vung Tau beach that was <u>not</u> OD green and brown. As I lay on my back on the hot sand, I cried. Somehow being in Vung Tau, away from the sights and sounds of the war, I was able to allow my tears to begin to flow — and flow they did for three days. Tears would roll from the outside corners of my eyes, down the side of my face and onto the sand. I realized what was happening and suddenly thought, *Oh my gosh! what if I do this when I*

---

[1] *365 Days,* Ronald J. Glasser M.D., George Braziller, Inc. 1980

*return to duty?* I could not afford that, because it meant the soldiers might see my tears and believe it meant they were going to die. I knew I had to do something. Long ago, when I first came to Vietnam, I put something there to stop the tears, but what could I do now? The answer crept up slowly and then popped into my awareness. *Build a wall.*

Over the next few days, gradually and methodically, I built a brick wall around my heart. I could feel myself doing it and see it being built. The wall was strong and I knew it would do its job. It held my heart tight so that it would not express intense emotions. It was as though I was steeled against feeling emotions. Mostly, it stopped me from feeling sadness and grief, horror and shock. It also left me numbed out again. Still, out on the sand and in the sun, I was finally able to relax and sleep. In fact, I slept a lot during those three days.

During my short stay in Vung Tau, I drank beer, ate pineapples and Chinese food, plus talked with the Aussies. Many were blonde, had easy-going personalities and laughed a lot. I loved to sit with them at dinner and listen to them tell me about Australia.

On the beach at Vung Tau, I soaked up the rays of the hot sun, took naps and ate the sweetest juiciest pineapples I had ever tasted. The Vietnamese women had a way of peeling and carving the pineapples so that I could hold the stalk and eat the upside-down, carved pineapple, whole. They were smaller than the ones I had eaten back home and it was easy to hold, like an ice cream cone to lick and suck the juice and nibble on the fruit. They were so juicy there was no stopping the flow as I constantly licked as fast as I could. I ate several every day. When I had devoured the pineapple and was lying in the hot sand, I began to relax. As I calmed my body and mind, I felt myself drifting back and remembering how I came to be here in Vietnam and in this war…

• • • • •

In 1966, I was hearing on the radio about a place called Vietnam. I didn't know where it was, or anything about the country or its people, but I did know that our American boys were going there to fight and they were only teenagers. America had called her young men to go to Vietnam to prevent a communist takeover. As I listened to the radio announcer, I flashed back to what I had said when I was nineteen sitting with my friends in the nursing school dorm: "If there is ever another war and I am single, I'll go." Now at twenty-six I asked myself, did I still mean that, and the answer was yes! My life was not going anywhere at the time, so I went to the recruiters. I was too short to be an air force flight nurse; I had to be five foot two inches and I was only five feet. The navy wanted me to serve for two years in a U.S Naval hospital before they would put me on a hospital ship, which is where I wanted to be. In my naïveté, I thought the war would be over in two years. The army recruiter said, "We really need operating room nurses," and they told me that I could go to school after Vietnam and get my degree on the GI bill. I thought that sounded pretty good, especially since I was already working on my degree part-time. So, I decided to join the Army Nurse Corps and had my swearing in ceremony with Jane Carson, the nurse recruiter. On the way back home after talking with the recruiters, I had one of those 'Aha' moments and recalled my blue-career booklet from age nine. My booklet showed me as a military nurse. I had pictures of nurses from each branch of the military that I had put together for the school assignment.

Within a month, I left Los Angeles where I had worked as a nurse for three years. In those three years I worked with medical and surgical patients, orthopedic patients, did intensive care and coronary care nursing, developed many friends and matured as a young woman exploring different cultures. I had grown up poor, had limited life experiences. I was a three -year- old on the streets by myself watching people. My dad was in the Army Air Corps during WWII after Pearl Harbor was bombed. I was two- years- old when that happened.

As I grew, the greatest support I received was at the lighthouse. It was blue and white and was within walking distance of the apartment where we lived. I would pour out my feelings there while looking at the light and talking to God. My uncle Will, who I loved, promised to send me to medical school. He died when I was in my second year of High

School and my friend who was a senior the previous year, left for college and I felt bereft. I had to let go of the dream to be a doctor and instead went to nursing school. After becoming a nurse, I felt rich and hungry to learn about other people, ideas, and cultures.

I took a few weeks off and headed home to Atlantic City, New Jersey to ready myself for my upcoming basic training. I had no idea what I might encounter, and, oh, boy, was I in for a surprise. From the moment I arrived in Fort Sam Houston, located just outside of San Antonio, Texas, I was immersed in so many different classes my head was spinning. There seemed to be army protocols for everything. In addition, I had to learn wound care, administration, ranks, how the system works, and the endless rules and regulations. We marched, drilled and learned to salute which we had a lot of practice doing. In order to go to or from the mess hall and the mailroom, we had to cross the quadrangle where we marched. It was a large open concrete square equivalent to a city block surrounded by buildings. When crossing it, we always met many soldiers and officers of either lower or higher rank. That meant saluting about twenty-five to fifty times each way. I started to go around and behind the buildings so that I was not constantly saluting across the quadrangle.

In the mornings, the nurses in basic training ate breakfast in a place called the Pit. It was down a few steps from street level, was very dark, smelled like booze and smoke, and always played loud rock and roll music. I loved that kind of music, but having the worst songs blasted loudly in that dark smelly place early in the morning was an assault on my ears and head. I hated going there.

While in basic training we were taught to do emergency cricothyroidotomies; putting a hole and then a tube into the front of the neck, trachea (windpipe), so that the person could breathe around an obstruction. We learned to rescue goats paralyzed by curare' by performing the cricothyroidotomy emergency surgery to save them. It had to be done quickly before they died. We used the same goats to learn how to debride wounds. Our task was to learn to identify which tissue, especially muscle, was living and which was dead. We removed all the dead tissue. Those goats gave their lives so we could learn how to save the lives of our brother soldiers.

The culmination of basic training was going to Camp Bullis, where we lived in tents and worked in tent hospitals under warlike conditions. We had simulated casualties; soldiers made up to appear wounded with tags on them describing the type of wound, and where it was located. We had to do triage[2], role-play surgery and care for them post-op.

At one point in basic training, we had 'familiarization with weapons,' and learned to load and fire a .45 pistol. Even though we were noncombatants and not issued a pistol, we needed to know how to load and shoot one should we need to defend our patients or ourselves. Some of the women acted out during these challenging moments; one of them held a gun to my head, laughed and said, "Oh don't worry, it is not loaded." It was not a time to play around. I was angry, grabbed the end of the pistol and turned it back toward the woman who was pointing it at my head telling her: "Not funny — do not point that at anyone unless you intend to shoot it."

After basic training, I was sent to Letterman General Hospital in San Francisco to attend the five-month operating nurse course. The hospital was located on the area known as the Presidio of San Francisco. The path to the OR took me down many long corridors and one in particular was lined with wounded Vietnam soldiers wearing bright blue pajamas sitting in wheelchairs, with a look in their eyes that became known as the thousand-yard stare. I felt like I was running the gauntlet. The only way to get to the OR was to walk down that corridor. Walking down it reminded me of walking down my street, New Hampshire Avenue, in Atlantic City, N.J., when I was only nine years old.

Back in Atlantic City, I would walk from home to the trolley, about four blocks. On the way, I would see a man in a wheelchair hunched over and drooling. I was afraid of him, so I would walk on the other side of the street — always sneaking a look at him so he could not see

---

[2] Sorting by priority re: severity of wound and chance of survival.

me looking. I would do this day after day, gathering my courage until finally I had enough courage to walk on his side of the street. Then, when I got close to him, I would walk very fast until I passed him. After about a week of doing that, I slowed down and worked up the courage to stop and talk to him. He was in a big, wooden, cane-backed wheelchair with big wheels on each side and he was wearing an old, worn, brown sweater. His chair was alongside a dark reddish-brown brick building. I would have to walk beside the chair to pass him. There was plenty of sidewalk to do that, but I was afraid he would try to grab me or something. I was afraid of everything when I was nine. I felt like I could die or that whatever happened to him was going to happen to me if he touched me. He started to call to me. His voice sounded like a whisper, "Hi little girl." I didn't answer on several of my faster and even slower walks by him.

Finally, one day I stopped and said, "Hi," and I really looked at him for the first time. He was not old, but he looked old. His arms were held close to his body in front of his stomach and chest, his hands were knotted and his shoulders sagged. He was alone, like me. His hands were tightly clenched, his face covered with stubbly hair and he had drool coming out of his mouth. His head looked down and it seemed hard for him to talk. I didn't stay very long that time. The next time, I stopped and stayed a little longer even though I still felt afraid of him.

One day the scare was gone. I don't know where it went, it just wasn't there anymore. He said, "I am lonely here in this chair and I am glad when you come by and talk to me."

"My name is Sarah, what is your name and what is wrong with you?"

"My name is Bobby. I was in a war and came back like this. My hands get tighter and tighter and hurt so much."

"Can I help you?"

"Yes," he said, "pull my hands open."

He guided me through how to open his hands. I put my little hands on one of his big hands with his palms up, I pulled his fingers down and out. I had to pull hard to get the fingers to come down and I had to keep doing it until they would stay open a little bit. When I could get them down and open for a minute, I would rub the palm of his hand, which was very soft. I stayed there and massaged his hands one at a time until they relaxed more and he felt better. To do this, I had to also pull his arms out a little, so they did not hug his body so tightly. I had to use my whole body weight to get his arms out from his body.

He liked chocolate and asked me to get him a chocolate bar. I did not have any money but he did, in his sweater pocket. I got the money out of his pocket and went to the store and bought him a Hershey Chocolate bar. He was unable to open it or even feed himself because of his contractures, so I had to feed it to him.

I began to look forward to seeing him and helping him and I would skip down the street to see him, even when I didn't have to go to the trolley. One day when I went down to see him, he wasn't there and I felt sad. I went again the next day and he wasn't there again. Again, and again I went, but he was never there. I think he died. I cried and cried because I missed my friend.

I remembered Bobby when I was walking down that long corridor at Letterman General Hospital in 1966, in my crisp white army nurse uniform. I remembered him because of the young men in wheelchairs watching me walk as fast as I could past them, because I didn't want to see, feel and know what they felt or experienced. Bobby was taken away; he was gone and no one knew where or why. I did not want to experience the pain of that kind of loss again.

I tried to walk fast and not look at the guys with their sad, pleading eyes, young handsome faces, and broken bodies. They sat in wheelchairs on both sides of that long corridor. There was no other way to get to the operating room (OR). I planned an extra ninety minutes, to walk down that corridor so I could talk with those soldiers. When they started to reach out to me with their eyes and their voices, I had to stop. I stopped and listened to their stories. Stories of a place called Vietnam — across many waters. I heard their voices tell me of war, of pain, and of people. One of the guys was only eighteen, had red hair, blue eyes and no legs. He lost his legs when he was riding in the back of a truck called a deuce and half. A nine-year-old Vietnamese girl threw a hand grenade into the back of the truck, and blew off his legs. His story was my first awareness that this Vietnam War was unfathomable. *How could that be? What did a nine-year old girl know of hand grenades, a tool of war?* My mind could not fathom how a little girl could be taught to kill by throwing a grenade. I was soon to be assailed by experiences beyond anything I knew, that were vile and gut wrenching. This young soldier, Red, was very brave and strong. He was not crying about his lost legs. He was focused only on his goal to walk on new legs, to stand tall and proud, and to be the best man he could be at his buddy's wedding.

As I got to know Red and some of the other guys better, I made time before and after my OR duty, to visit with them and hear about their physical therapy (PT) and their progress. It was a painstakingly slow process of getting used to wearing an artificial limb, building up the strength of the stump to bear weight and to toughen up the skin. The skin of the stump is not as tough as the soles of our feet, which holds our weight normally. It took stamina, physical and emotional strength, to bear the daily pain and work of rehabilitation. Red was up to the task. He worked hard, sweated, swore, and occasionally cried. We became friends. What he wanted most was for me to help him walk on his artificial legs. I agreed to help him.

Meanwhile in the five-month operating room course, I learned everything about being an OR nurse on any type of case from orthopedics to urology, general surgery, thoracic, gynecological and C-sections, head and neck, neurosurgery, facial, eyes, ears, nose, and throat (EEENT) and even open-heart surgery. I not only knew the anatomy and physiology for all systems and areas of the body, I knew the various types of surgical procedures and what to anticipate in sequence during an operation. In that way, I could anticipate what instruments the surgeon would need and have them ready. What the OR course could not prepare me for —were the horrors of war wounds.

On neurosurgery cases, the patient was often sitting up on a specially designed table that held them in a sitting position with their head braced. The OR table had to be up pretty high because the patient was sitting up, which meant I had to walk up several steps to reach the very high long wide table we worked from. The table was three feet by four feet, because it held so many instruments and needed items, including the drill to make holes in the skull bone. I didn't like doing neurosurgery because I did not appreciate feeling like I was on the ceiling for hours working on that very high table. It was very tedious and my own body cringed every time they drilled holes in the skull.

I was one of the few from the OR course who scrubbed in on open-heart surgery cases. I liked them because they were active and I had a lot to do. I had to be alert all the time. We also used the heart lung machine and I liked having the opportunity to help repair hearts. The part of open-heart surgery that I could have done without, was the surgeon who thought he had the right to molest me. He was the open-heart specialist who came around behind me when his part of the case was done and the other surgeon was closing the chest. I was still scrubbed in (wearing sterile gown and gloves). This big man, the colonel, put his hands under my sterile outer gown and grabbed my breasts from behind me. I was stunned and shocked and could not speak at first. I had never seen or heard about military sexual assault/harassment before, did not like it and was not willing to experience it. He was a colonel and I was only a first lieutenant. We were in an army hospital and he did outrank me. I thought about that, but I also knew that no matter what his rank or how good a surgeon he was, he had no right to touch me like that if I did not consent. In my strongest voice I said, "colonel, if you don't take your hands off me right now, I will break scrub and report you to the chief nurse!" He was out the door in a heartbeat and never touched me again. I was also never assigned to any of his cases after that. The head nurse told me the next day that I was not permitted in his operating room ever again because I was insubordinate to him. Did that mean I was supposed to just let him do as he pleased with me? I had heard the phrase 'rank has its privileges' but certainly molesting me or any other nurse was not a given privilege. (My previous book explores this: *Women Under Fire: Abuse in the Military www.womenunderfire.net*)

As the end of the OR course was drawing near, I received my orders to report for duty in Vietnam on January 16, 1967. At that point I was well trained, had been in the army over six months, and had learned a lot more about the Vietnam War, none of which was very positive. I began to have an attitude. If someone was not happy with me, or something I was doing or saying, my response was, "So what are you going to do, send me to Vietnam?"

My attitude, however, was very different with the patients. They were like my brothers who had been hurt in that war and I was gentle loving and supportive with them. I listened intently when they shared feelings or experiences with me. I did small things to help them if they needed it. I encouraged them in PT, especially when they were discouraged by their slow progress. Some did not have use of their arms or hands so I helped them write letters if they needed that.

The date of Red's buddy's wedding was in December. Red was working hard to be ready. The day of the wedding, a group of his buddies along with me, all drove him to the wedding site. We discovered that we would have to go up a very steep flight of stairs to get to the apartment where the ceremony was being held. We put Red in his wheelchair and the guys lifted him and his chair all the way up the steps. He was nervous because he also knew he could only stand with balance for about five minutes. Red was able to stay in his wheelchair for the first part of the ceremony, me sitting on his one side, his buddy on the other. When his moment finally came, we helped him up, but made sure to let him find his own balance, knowing how important that was to him. We stood beside him as he did his part in the ceremony. Sweat poured off him as he stood there so very proud in his full class A uniform. He was truly the Best Man he could be, and showed that to all. I was very happy to support him and help him do that before I left San Francisco. I completed the OR course, said goodbye to Red and his buddies and went home on leave to prepare for my journey to Vietnam. *What could I take with me? What would I need to sustain me while I was there? How do I prepare for something I have never experienced?* I knew I would take a duffel bag, a footlocker, and my ukulele in its case. I had a baritone ukulele, larger than those most commonly known and not as big as a guitar. I knew that I would need to play music to express my feelings and myself while I was in Vietnam.

I have always used a musical instrument to express my feelings from the time I was very young. In those days, not quite even knowing what I was doing and how it helped me, when my family would argue, I would pound on the piano, imitating what I was hearing and feeling.

In my duffel bag, I packed all my uniforms, fatigues, boots, poncho, field jacket, OD army issue underwear and towels. My footlocker was full of small boxes of All soap, (because you can wash in cold water with it), and a few civilian clothes, a pair of sneakers, pajamas, pictures, tampons, and books.

My trip to Vietnam began from Travis Air Force base, not far from San Francisco. The terminal was filled with hundreds of women and men in military uniforms heading for Vietnam. I could feel the intense anxiety and fear all around in the large room. Everyone was dealing with their feelings in different ways. Some were loud and laughing, some were quiet saying nothing, while others were pacing. I was leaning against a wall observing and being quiet. After about two hours, I climbed aboard a World Airways jet, in my summer green cord uniform with about 199 other nurses in summer green cords. We chattered and chittered, our anxieties all a flutter, as the stewardesses fed us around the clock. Literally, we were fed every four hours. The look in their eyes said: "You are courageous, I couldn't do what you are doing, here eat you may never get to eat again."

We landed in Alaska first where it was eleven degrees. I was wearing my summer short-sleeve uniform and paper-thin raincoat. I was freezing, trembling, teeth chattering, trying to think hot. We had to stay in a hangar with no heat for what seemed like hours. Finally, we got back on the plane and I gradually stopped shaking from being so very cold. They fed us again and then turned out all the lights so we could sleep. A few hours later they woke us up again — that's right, to eat.

Next, we landed in Japan to refuel where it was a warm twenty-one degrees, but at least we were inside a building with some heat. I guess they decided since we were going to be hot for a year in Vietnam to let us experience cold first.

During the previous four months, from September to December of 1967, there had been passionate demonstrations on college campuses...the burning of draft cards and the American flag, along with general anti-military protests. I was shocked by all of it. My dad, my brother and two uncles were all veterans. All the services were represented in my family. My dad was in the Army Air Force Signal Corps in WWII, one uncle was a Marine from WWII and the other had been in the Navy. My brother was in the Army during the Cold War as a helicopter crew chief. Here I was in an army hospital with guys who fought for the cause of freedom and were wounded doing that. I felt angry and resentful of the demonstrations. I was glad to be getting out of the United States where it seemed so many were acting un-American.

# Chapter 2
# UP CLOSE AND PERSONAL IN VIETNAM – PART 1

When we landed at Bien Hoa Air Base and I exited the plane, I was hit in the face by a wave of oppressive heat. With the heat came a smell that I lived with for a full year. It was always in the air and went right up into my nostrils to let me know I was now in Vietnam. That smell was a combination of sweat, dirt, dead flesh, people, excrement of all types and the firepower of war.

Once on the airfield, an officer welcomed us, "In country." He told us, "We have planned a special hello for you in the air." I heard the sounds first and then looked up to see some jets screaming and screeching through the skies above; they dipped their wings, rolled over, and flew in a circle above us.

It was a moment of excitement before we were given the order to find our duffle bags. I looked behind the plane that brought us to see 200 OD duffle bags, a few of which had colored ribbons on them to make them stand out. Those who had the wisdom to put a ribbon on their bag found them easily and quickly. In the blistering heat, I searched and searched for my bag; sweat poured off my whole body, drenching my uniform, rolling down my nose and the sides of my face. I looked at each identical bag, reading the black letters to find the one with my name and serial number. It seemed to take forever. Each of the

100 plus nurses was searching ceaselessly for their own bags. Once I found mine, I was whisked off in an OD army bus with heavy crisscross wire fencing covering the windows. I innocently asked, "Why the wire," only to hear, "This is a war zone, Ma'am, it's to keep out the grenades."

"Oh," I said timidly and promptly felt both stupid and scared. The bus took me down a long dusty road from the Bien Hoa Airbase to the 90th Replacement Battalion at Long Binh, a place where I would learn so much about this country – its people, their unique language, money, and, of course, the mosquitoes and malaria pills.

When we arrived, we were taken to a large room where the Chief Nurse of Vietnam, Colonel Anna Mae Hays, was to address us. As I stood there, still sweating from my duffle bag adventure, I noticed a young nurse across the room. She was obviously just out of school, and was as terrified as anyone I'd ever seen. Her skin was white and she was shaking and crying. I learned that she was assigned to the 12th Evacuation Hospital and was frightened to go there because it was in the Iron Triangle.[3] I was assigned to Pleiku, the 71st Evacuation Hospital, which was in I Corps, (Military Region one comprising ten different units, pronounced eye corps) close to the demilitarized zone (DMZ) and the North. The 71st was being built and was not yet completed, so I was reassigned to the 67th Evacuation Hospital at Qui Nhon, on the coast of the South China Sea. Qui Nhon was a slower, easier place to be. I heard the nurses there took care of a lot of Vietnamese civilians. I went to comfort the terrified young nurse and discovered that she had the same military occupational specialty[4] (MOS) as I had. She too was an OR nurse. Seeing her terror and feeling my own desire to serve young American GI's, I offered to switch with her. She was immediately relieved, grateful, and stopped shaking and crying. Together we went to the Chief Nurse and proposed the switch in assignments. Because of the young nurse's obvious terror and her

---

[3] The Iron Triangle was an area of land between Tay Ninh, Saigon and Bien Hoa. The area encompasses the Hobo woods and Cu Chi. It was in III (three) Corps.
[4] The specific job we did in the military designated by letters and numbers.

MOS being the same, the Chief Nurse agreed to the switch; now I would be going to the 12th Evacuation Hospital at Cu Chi.

That night in the officers' club I met two guys who were my drill sergeants in basic training. They were both dust-off pilots[5] who asked, "Where will you be stationed?"

I proudly told them, "The 12th Evac at Cu Chi." There was silence as they looked at each other, and their faces went from light to dark.

Sergeant Phillips said, "You don't want to go there. Can you change it?"

"Why?" I asked. They told me that the 12th Evac was the worst place I could go because most of the fighting was right there in the Iron Triangle. That was where all the offensive action was focused and there were a lot of Viet Cong[6] (VC) there. The 12th was the busiest hospital in Vietnam in 1967. They took care of soldiers from both sides and civilians.

Sergeant Phillips said, "The nurses are not safe there and their base-camp is under fire from VC mortars almost weekly." I did feel scared and tensed up when he told me all that and I saw how fearful he looked. I had some trepidation for the moment but I had no intention of changing my assignment. That is where I was most needed so that is where I would go. Deep down, I knew I was challenging God, and now, more than ever, with the sergeant's warning still ringing in my ears, I wanted to know the reason or purpose for me being in this life.

Going from the 90th replacement battalion to the 12th Evac Hospital was my first helicopter ride. I looked at the large OD helicopter and saw that there were no doors on it; I was shocked. I looked at the row of nylon seats I was to sit on with great trepidation. I chose the middle seat because I didn't want to be by the open door. This chopper had two wide-open sides with no visible or actual shelter, and flying low through

---

[5] Dust-offs were the helicopters designated to pick up and deliver casualties to hospitals. They were given the name because of their rotor blades 'dusting off' the helipad.

[6] Viet Cong were the enemy of the republic of South Vietnam and fought in black pajamas. They were referred to as guerillas and were part of the communist regime led by Ho Chi Minh, in the North.

jungle in the middle of a war zone without something, anything that remotely seemed like protection, seemed crazy to me. I was at least not going to be right by the opening, even though it was clear that if we were hit, it did not much matter where I was sitting. I was frightened and excited at the same time. The guys flying the Huey told me one horror story after another about troops caught in a cross-fire, being blown up by landmines or rocket propelled grenades called RPGs, and being overrun and ambushed. As we descended to the helipad at the 12th Evacuation Hospital, they told me to pick up my stuff. It was a short ten-minute ride, both noisy and windy. They pointed to the Quonset huts that made up the 12th Evacuation Hospital, and told me to jump. I was stunned, puzzled, and in disbelief!

"You gotta be kidding me – put this thing down!" I shouted, trying my best to be heard above the growl of the rotor blades.

But they would not set the chopper down, and instead, hovered about six feet over the helipad. I was going to have to jump. All five feet tall, 100 pounds of me wearing fatigues and boots, carrying a brown leather instrument case and having to jump out of a helicopter six feet off the ground. It must have been an initiation of some kind. My heart was pounding almost as loud as the chuff chuff blade sounds. I kept pointing down and saying the word, "down" and they shook their heads no. I did not seem to have a choice, so I took a deep breath, bent my knees a few times and then jumped. I landed pretty solid, with a jolt to my knees and spine, but I was OK. Then I looked up and they were going up and away. I yelled up at them as they lifted away, "Where do I go?" They pointed. I walked on the desolate barren red/yellow dirt amongst the gray Quonset huts that were all lined up in two rows about one hundred yards apart.

I walked in the direction the guys had pointed to find the headquarters building. There I met the executive officer. He was a strac[7]

---

[7] Shined boots plus the appearance of a proud, competent trooper who can be depended on for excellent performance in any circumstance.

looking guy with his fatigues pressed and starched. I said, "Lt. Blum reporting for duty, Sir!" and saluted. Pretty strac of me, I thought.

He pointed to my ukulele case and asked, "What is that?"

"It is a machine gun, Sir," I said smiling, "I thought I might need it over here." He did not think it was funny and spent the next ten minutes letting me know that. "Lt. Blum you are being disrespectful and insubordinate to the executive officer of this hospital.

I expect you to be respectful of me and any other officer of higher rank while you are here. Do you understand?" He lectured me in his tirade about respect for commanding officers. I got the message; don't joke with him.

He told me to report to the chief nurse of the hospital and I did. She told me where I would bunk, where I would work and then told me to get settled in before I reported for duty. *How do I settle in when I don't have my stuff yet?* What I didn't know at the time was that it would be coming by truck a few hours later and would be unceremoniously dumped in the middle of the dirt compound between the rows of buildings. In the meantime, I looked at my space, which consisted of a metal bed with a mattress beside the wooden outside wall. There were two-by-fours running horizontal about head high along the outside wall and three interior partitions made of bamboo screening between the areas to my right and left and one in front. There was an opening that served as the door with long beaded bamboo strands hanging from the doorjamb to give some cover for the door opening. This was to be home for a year. Uh oh!

I found some guys who told me I needed to scrounge[8] building materials. They told me what that meant, where to go and how to do it. So, I scrounged. I ended up with wood, nails, a hammer and a piece of Masonite. With no knowledge or skill to speak of, I was in the back of my hooch,[9] making shelves. I looked at the pieces of wood and tried them out in different ways before I started pounding nails. I had to figure out how to put them together and make them hold. I prayed over

---

[8] Looking for supplies and asking people where to find the things I needed.
[9] Name for our living quarters e.g., nurse's hooch

them to make sure they would stay together for a year. "Dear God, please help me get through this war and bless my shelves so they stay together for the year." Picture of me with my shelves behind

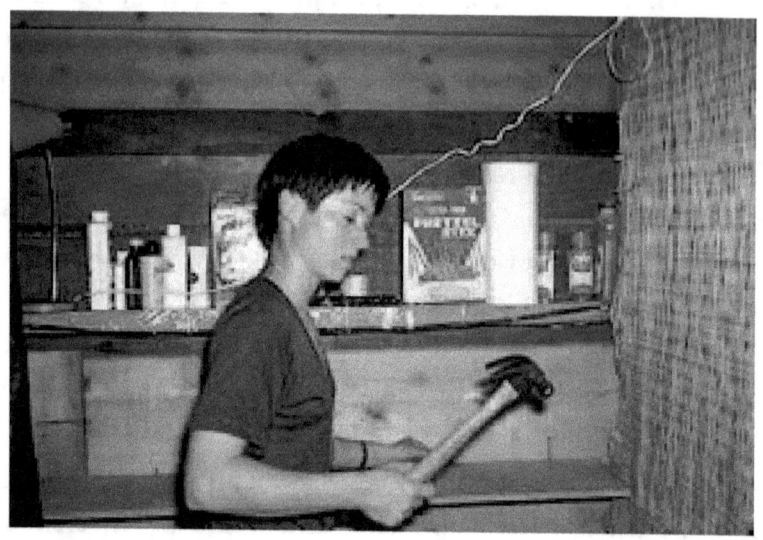

My shelves turned out looking mighty funny, but they worked and they did hold together for a year. In fact, I gave them to my replacement at the end of the year. When my duffel bag and footlocker came, I arranged everything in my hooch. My footlocker was filled with clothes, soap and girl-things. I used the shelves for books and later, canned goods and supplies from the PX (post exchange/store). I put my family pictures on the top shelf.

I scrounged a large cardboard box that held heavy equipment. It looked like a box that at home a refrigerator might come in. I cut the front in half horizontally so that it could be a door. I made it work with a piece of string. The box was a closet that I could open and close; then I put in a horizontal pole to hold my clothes. I put my civilian clothes and field jacket in the closet and my helmet on top of it. I avoided wearing my helmet as much as I could. Later, on one of my very few trips into the village of Cu Chi, I added a big washbasin on top, purchased in Cu Chi and paid with Vietnamese money. The army did not want us to go into the village because it was dangerous and we nurse's, had a price on our heads. If captured, we were worth $10,000 American Dollars.

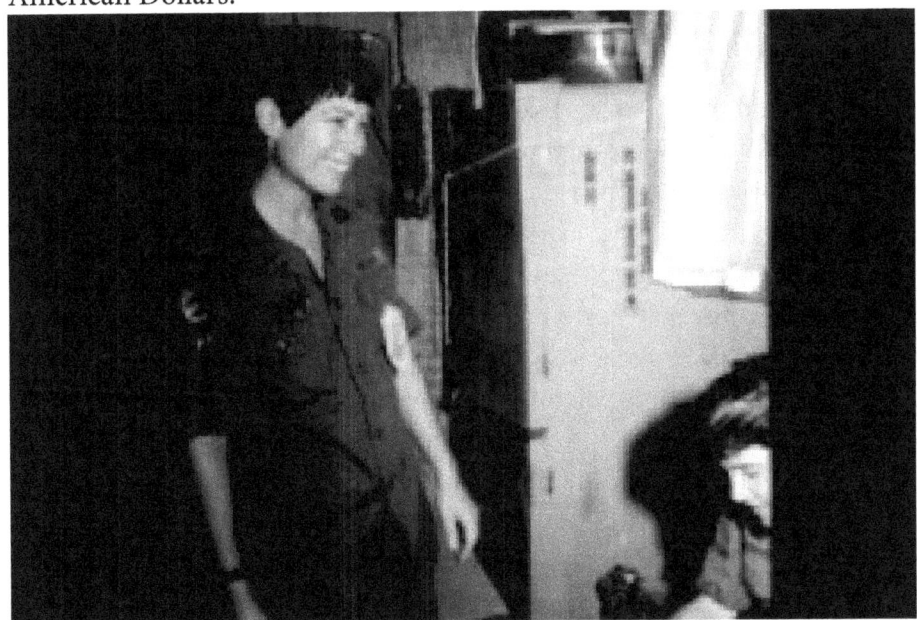

4. Me with Claire sitting on my foot locker and my cardboard closet between us. The nurses had three hooches side by side and behind them were our latrines, (outhouses) water cans and where we could hang laundry. (Back of my hooch/latrine)

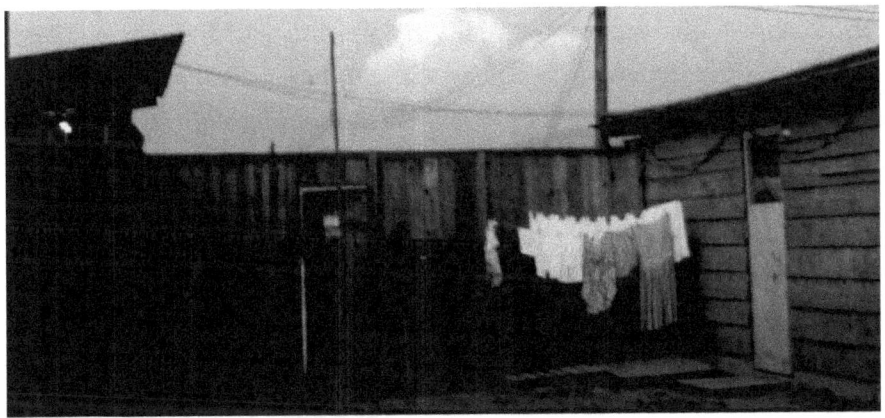

5. Back of our hooch with laundry drying beside water cans with latrine on left.

My work at the 12th Evac Hospital in surgery was pretty intense and grueling. The helicopters brought in the casualties on OD canvas stretchers soaked in their blood. The casualties went directly to pre-op, a Quonset hut where they did triage. The pilot of the chopper would radio ahead to pre-op and say they were on their way, their estimated time of arrival (ETA) and how many and what type of casualties. When the casualties were off-loaded, they were brought right into triage and sorted by injury. The worst casualties with the greatest chance of survival went first and then in degrees after that, next worst with the greatest chance of living. Those that were so bad they were expected to die were called expectant. They were left in pre-op and a nurse stayed with them until they died. At our hospital, our nurses and doctors didn't put many guys into the expectant category because we believed we could save most of them. When I say we, I include myself, because it was an overall belief, even though I was not assigned to pre-op. I am sure that there were times we made choices that were not the best. When there was a difficult choice to make and many casualties, we had to sort according to the strict military guidelines. That meant, to not use precious resources on a casualty who would probably die anyway, while others who could live had to wait and get worse. In pre-op, they tore or cut off the soldier's fatigues and boots, examined all their wounds and decided in what order they came to us in the OR. Next photo shows off-loading a casualty from a dust-off helicopter. Dust-off/Medivac is the name given to the chopper with the red cross on them indicating they were noncombatants. Chopper blades cause dust/dirt to move, so they nicknamed them "dust-off."

• • • • •

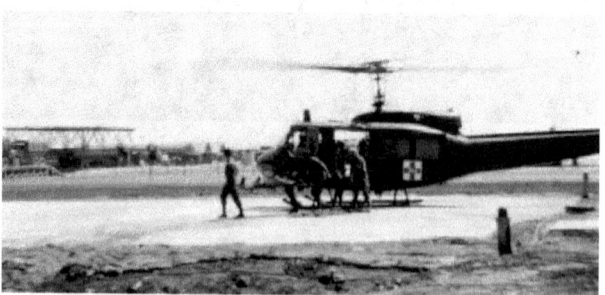

6. Medivac chopper off-loading a casualty on our helipad.

Reliving those memories of being assigned to the OR, and those first days at the 12th Evac Hospital, hit me like a thump on my chest, and I shot up from the sand, my heart pounding, sweat all over my body. My mind in shock, it took several breaths to realize that I was still lying on the warm welcoming beach at Vung Tau, supposedly taking in some needed R&R. I had gone back to the memory of my first days at the 12th Evac and understood in that moment, that I had to return. I would have to go back to the OR the next day and I wasn't ready emotionally. I knew what I had to do, so focused again on the brick wall of protection around my heart. I was determined to return to the 12th Evac OR and do my best to fulfill my mission. I had to stop being vulnerable and be tougher skinned. I couldn't let it all get to me. There had to be a way.

I had dinner with the Aussies and asked them for ideas. They truly did not comprehend the depth, breadth and intensity of what I saw, heard and felt for hours and hours of every day and the impact it was having on me. Their answers were to drink more and laugh more. I know I did more drinking when I got back, I am not sure I was able to laugh more.

Once I was back in the operating room, I went into action. I was usually a scrub nurse, meaning I scrubbed my hands and arms up to my elbows in Betadine for five-Ten minutes then put on a sterile gown and gloves. I was either working with the surgeon and handing him instruments, or I was doing the same thing the surgeon was doing or some of both. When I did the same thing as the surgeon, it was usually on cases where the soldier had hit a landmine and had pellet wounds all over his body. The surgeon would come in scrubbed, look at the patient and ask me, "Do you want the right or left side?" and we would go to work. In those cases, we made a clean cut over each pellet wound with a scalpel. Then we opened it gradually and cut away all the dead tissue. To test muscle, we used forceps to see if it moved, if it did then it was alive. If it did not move, it was dead and we cut it out. Often, we could tell the difference by the color. The redder the muscle the more likely it was alive. The very dark muscle was not. We cut away all the dead tissues and looked for the metal. We removed the metal pellets with forceps and put them in a metal basin, so we were constantly hearing the 'clink' sound of metal hitting metal. There were more times than I could remember when we filled those basins working on just one patient. After we took out the metal and dead tissues, we washed the wounds over and over with sterile saline solution.[10]

In cases where I was both nurse and surgeon, I did everything as nurse with my right hand that I normally would do with two hands, and the left hand was holding a retractor to hold open the chest or belly. Threading needles with one hand was the hardest task. The way I made it work was to put the needle in a hemostat clamp with the eye facing up and then put the thread through with my one free hand. I would also cut blood vessel ties for the main surgeon or put my finger on the catgut[11] so the surgeon could get a good tie.

The doctors were all different but most were very cynical. They didn't want to be there, hated the situation and the lack of good equipment and supplies. They were good surgeons, did a great job and they became better and better as time went on. Only a few remained resentful. We all learned to work well together under pressure and keep our esprit de corps. One of our surgeons would have temper tantrums, throwing the catgut on the floor if we did not give it to him in his "preferred" way. He always expected us to cut the full length of the catgut into thirds, handing him one-third at a time to wrap around and tie-off a blood vessel. If we did what he asked for, he would have wasted about half of each package, which was totally unacceptable given our situation. We had packages of 3.0 catgut, yellow looking translucent sinew used to tie off bleeding blood vessels. Because we were constantly using it and had limited supplies, we would wind it around a small piece of sterile rubber tubing for each case. For our surgeon with the temper tantrums, I would hold up the rolled catgut to his face and say, "This is all the catgut you have for this case. You throw it and you're done!"

I could sympathize with the doctors. They were dedicated and spent years getting educated, trained, and prepared for a career as a surgeon, yet before they could establish themselves in the civilian medical world

---

[10] Salt solution that is isotonic i.e., in balance with the body.
[11] Suture material used to literally tie around the cut end of blood vessels so that they do not keep bleeding.

the U.S. Army drafted them. The doctors were told they would be serving their country by helping wounded soldiers for the next year in Vietnam. They were in a war they did not believe in, in the worst possible conditions and asked to do what, in many cases, seemed impossible. We truly saved lives in Vietnam that in any other previous war would have been lost. The helicopter changed everything. Wounded soldiers could be on the table within minutes of being wounded.

Corpsmen in the OR were enlisted guys who learned to be surgical technicians and also had to do guard duty. They were young sensitive guys trying to do a good job with what they were given to do. Their job was to circulate between the rooms and give us what we needed. The things the enlisted techs would give us were likely to be suture material, instruments, fresh gloves, saline solution, etc. They would open the wrapper, and either drop the contents onto our work-table or we would take it. They held the unsterile outside part and we would touch only the sterile parts inside the wrapper.

The nurses were diverse and came from different parts of the U.S., each with their own way of being, speaking and working. Claire was my best buddy. We talked about our feelings, the ugliness of war, and wished together that one-eyed Moshe Dyan[12] could lead us, so that our war could be over in six days, like the Israeli war that he led. She and I could talk about everything and laugh or cry together.

The operating room, where I was assigned, was a Quonset hut like the other wards. It had pale aqua painted wooden partitions between the individual sections. Each section had an operating room table, a seat at the head of the table for the anesthetist and all their equipment. For my use, there was a rectangular shaped low stainless-steel table that held all the instruments and supplies, a basin filled with water, an over-the-table tray on wheels, called a Mayo stand, that we used during the surgery to hand instruments and sutures to the surgeon. Our suture supplies were in small drawers in front of one partition beside a low table with paper and pen for reports. Along the outside wall was a shelf that housed extra supplies and instruments.

---

[12] Israeli Minister of Defense 1967.

In the last picture you can see me shaving the soldier's hair off his legs and the many pellet wounds from a land mine on them. I would have to cut each one open, take out the metal and drop it in the basin, cut out the dead tissue and irrigate the wound. Only after wound cleansings at the end do we bandage the wounds.

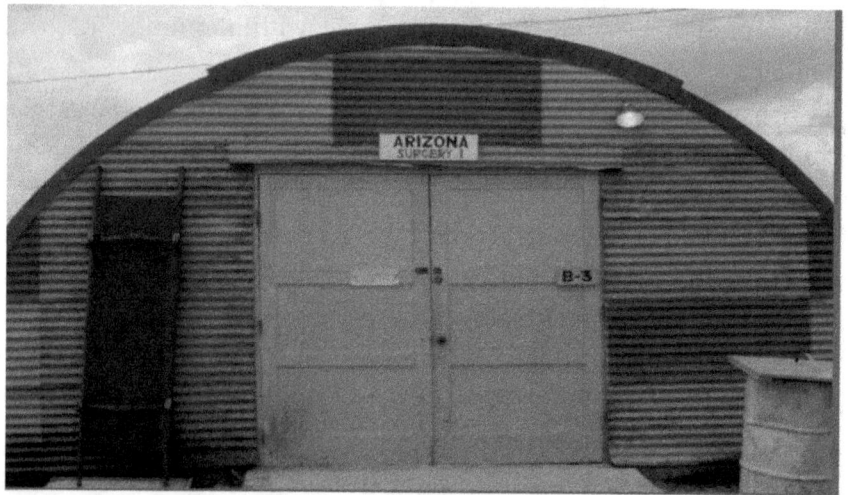

7. Main surgical unit. A second one was beside it that we used for overflow and it had a small area for nurses to rest.

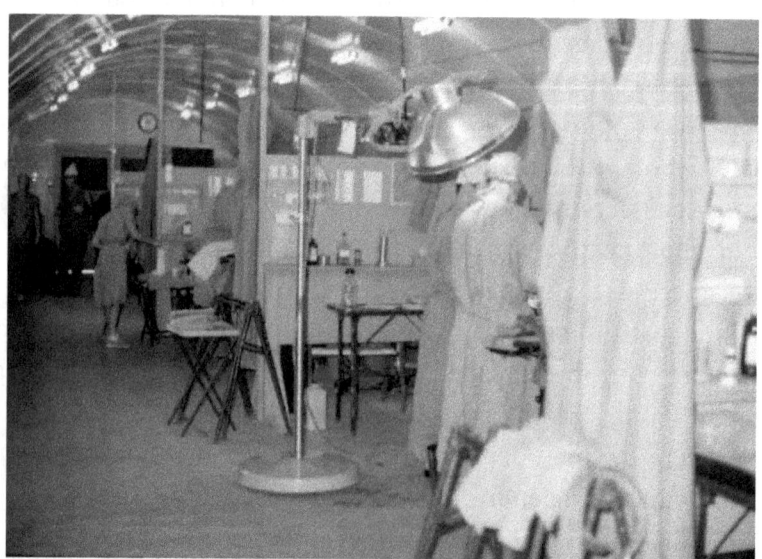

8. Inside the main operating room showing the individual spaces with operating tables, supplies etc. I am at far end in front of two technicians.

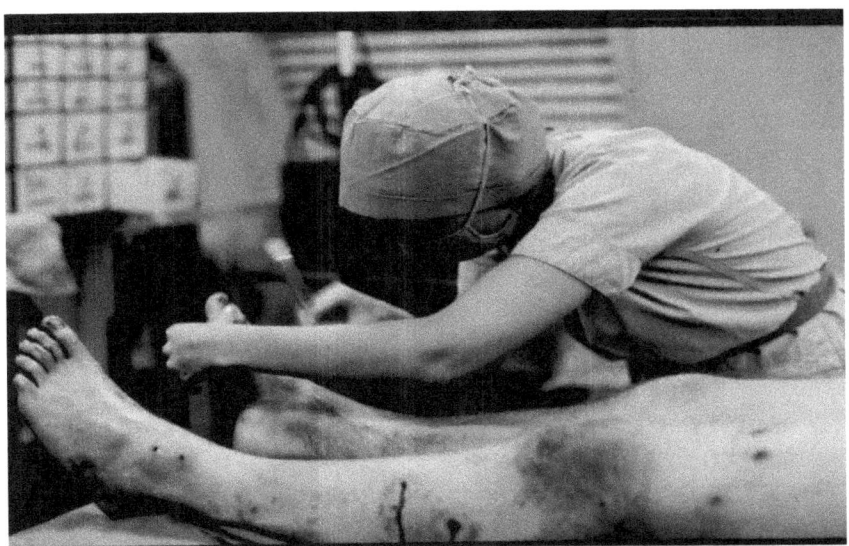

9. Me during a case shaving the soldier's hair off his legs, many pellet wounds on his legs, and suture drawers in background.

Overall, the hospital had two rows of Quonset huts starting on the B side, with headquarters, lab, x-ray and triage, our two operating room Quonsets and then recovery, plus B-6 and B-7. On the other side of the dry desolate dirt (not earth but dirt) between the B and C ramp, were the C wards housing the ill soldiers and those recovering from surgeries after the first forty-eight hours, including the POW and malaria wards.

We were called an evacuation hospital but functioned as a surgical hospital. The surgical hospitals were smaller and more mobile, could be packed up and moved in twenty-four hours. Soldiers brought to a surgical hospital could stay only long enough to have surgery, be stabilized and have their sutures removed. Then they would go to a longer stay hospital like an evacuation hospital, which are considered semi-mobile; the insides can be packed up and moved in forty-eight hours, but not the external buildings. Due to our location in relation to the fighting, wounded soldiers coming to us could not stay longer than four or five days because we had so many constantly coming in.

At age twenty-six, I was not prepared to see what I saw, or feel the depths of despair that I felt daily. Nineteen-year-old young men who could have been my brother or a boyfriend lost their legs, arms, eyes, had their guts shot to hell, their chests blown open or their faces or heads mutilated. The worst was a face that was half gone, which I couldn't look at. What kind of nurse am I that I cannot look at such a horror without being violently ill?

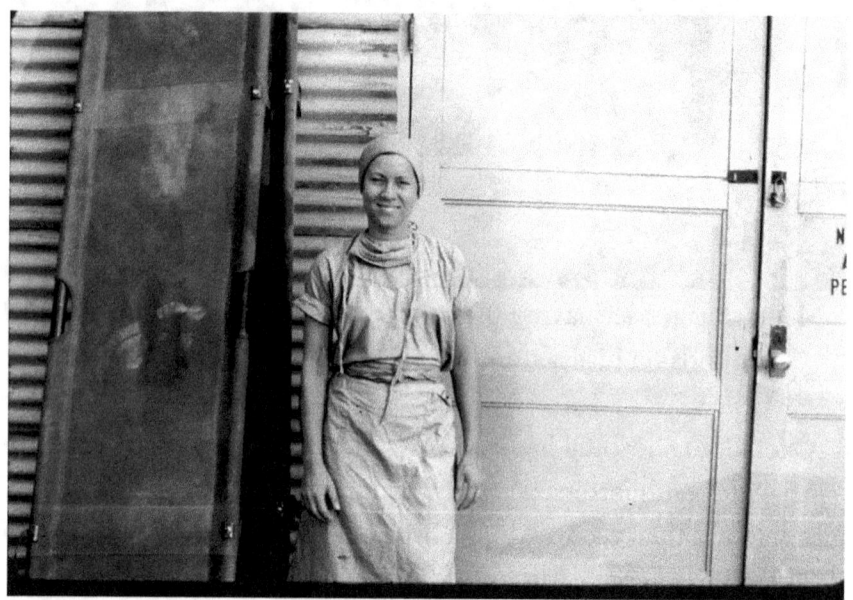

10. This picture was taken after working twenty hours on mass casualties.

The casualties came unceasingly. I never knew any of their names or what happened to them. One guy, whose memory haunts me, lost two legs, one arm and one eye. It was so painful to see these wonderful, innocent guys all mangled and maimed and not even know why, or have the "why" make any sense.

Day after day, chopper after chopper, brought more and more of these young men, doing a job they didn't want to do — kill. And who were they to kill? The enemy, VC soldiers, kids ages thirteen to nineteen. It was a kids' war. We couldn't tell who was and who was not VC, which made it all the harder to deal with.

After being there less than one month, we were hit by a mortar attack. Mortars came in from somewhere outside the base camp while I was in the shower. I heard sounds like a whistle, a thud and an explosion. It sounded ominous but I did not know the experience of mortars and wasn't sure what I was hearing until a young soldier wearing a flak jacket and helmet came into the hooch and said, "Everybody into the bunker!" He heard the shower and came by to tell me to go to the bunker. Our shower had no door, only two wooden partitions and the outside wall so he could see all of my naked body.

"I am all soaped up, I'll go when I get rinsed and dried off," I said.

He yelled, "Ma'am, if you don't go to the bunker right now, I will carry you there!" His intensity told me he meant it, so I went soapy and slipping down the hooch in my flip-flops and out into the bunker in my short little robe. My robe barely covered me to my buttocks. I was terrified when I shut the water off and heard those whistling sounds followed by a great loud thud and explosion. The bunker was dark. I went from the bright sunlight into the darkness. Fortunately, someone grabbed my hand to guide me knowing I was blinded momentarily. After a while my eyes adjusted. Most everyone had on army fatigues and flak jackets. Some nurses had on robes and muumuus.

A male voice said, "Hello," beside me and I almost jumped out of my skin because I thought there were only females in the bunker. I had only my skimpy robe on, more like a long shirt, which barely covered my wet soapy skin. I kept trying to cover up and felt embarrassed.

I could see my chief nurse across from me on a bench. She said, "When the all-clear sounds we will go back to what we were doing."

No sooner had she said that when a soldier popped his head into the bunker and said, "We need Lt. Blum in the OR right now!" I looked over at her and she nodded at me to go. First, I went back to the shower to rinse off the soap and the mud I now had on my feet and legs, then scrambled into my fatigues and boots and ran over to the O.R.

As I ran a zig zag course from my hooch to the OR, to try to avoid being hit by the incoming mortars, I heard soldiers yelling at me to put on my helmet and flak jacket. I did not wear them because I weighed only 100 pounds and with those on, I was more like 130 pounds and could not run as fast or well. That was the day I knew that I could easily die in Vietnam — and when I first experienced mass casualties while being under attack.

We had a steady stream of casualties all day and most of the evening. The choppers brought them in and went back for more. We had dust-offs coming in regularly; those are the helicopters with the red-cross in white background to designate them as noncombatants flying wounded only. There were also the Little Bears and Diamondheads, from the 25th Aviation Battalion[13] that were stationed down the road on our base-camp. The helicopters that brought in the casualties were usually Hueys. Dust-offs were designed for carrying casualties and the others were support helicopters from local units, which usually transported soldiers to combat areas. They often brought in guys from the 25th Infantry Division who were wounded. Units of the First Infantry Division[14] were also in our area and some from the 101st Airborne Division.

Most of the soldiers we saw had either lost body parts, had them blown up or blown off, or they had been hit by machine gun fire, AK 47s, grenades, landmines or stepped into or on a booby trap. Seeing the effects of all these on our guys was something I would never forget. My first "in country" training at Cu Chi was to attend the Landmine Booby Trap Education Center, where we saw all the types of booby traps, landmines, weapons and grenades they knew about and we even learned about tunnel[15] openings.

---

[13] *Angel's Wing*, by Joe Finch is one Little Bear's story of the 25th Aviation Battalion.
[14] We Were Soldiers is a movie that shows the infantry and helicopter connection, along with the attitudes in our military and government toward those of us serving in Vietnam.
[15] Tunnels of Cu Chi, is a book that describes the tunnels and the activities there.

Imagine a young healthy nineteen-year-old who has his whole life ahead of him. He is someone's brother, son, husband, father, friend, cousin, uncle, and beloved. He hears the call of his country to fight in Vietnam, or he is drafted and lands in a foreign country all alone until he finds the unit he is assigned to. He's there two weeks when he goes out on patrol and two hours into it, he steps on a hidden landmine losing his right leg, his left foot and has pellet wounds all over the lower half of his body. The unit would radio for a dust-off helicopter and within ten minutes he was on the OR table and we were clamping off bleeding ends of blood vessels, cleaning up the stumps surgically and removing all the pellets and dead tissue caused by those pellets and their velocity.

We washed out all his wounds thoroughly with saline before he left the OR. We washed war wounds a lot in the OR, and then on the wards after surgery. After the wounds are thoroughly washed, we would bandage them and send them to post-op. In post-op the nurses would watch him, check his vital signs, give him antibiotics, pain medications and every four hours they would soak off all his bandages, wash his wounds with saline, and rebandage them. When we were done with him, we took off the bloody sheets and put them in the dirty laundry basket, washed down the OR tables and trays with alcohol, and we mopped the blood off the floor. Then we got the next casualty and the next and the next. We were focused and didn't hear the choppers or the mortars fall. We just kept on working.

One day during my first two months in Vietnam my chief nurse, Major Molly Cicerchia, called me in to tell me several nurses were invited to a General's party. She told me we would be taken there by helicopter and that we could wear civilian clothes. When I talked with the other nurses they said, "It will be fun and we get to eat good food (as opposed to army food) and have real plates, silverware and glasses, instead of the plastic trays and the cups we use in the mess hall." I decided to go with them. We were picked up by a major and took, what he called the champagne flight, because he had a Styrofoam cooler in the helicopter filled with cups and champagne, which we drank on the way. When we arrived at the 3rd Surgical Hospital at Bien Hoa, there was a table set up with wonderful food, lots of salads, shrimp, Jell-O, and breads. It was some of the best food I had in Vietnam all year. The reason for the party was a birthday celebration for the General of the 198th Light Infantry Brigade. I met him and some other Generals too. They drank until they were drunk.

The General that was leading the First Infantry Division was behaving in a way that was disgusting to me. He was sticking cigarettes in his nose and ears, had slurred speech, and was being obnoxious when he grabbed me, put me on his lap and in his slurry words said, "You can be my girl and I will send for you when I want you and I am in a secure area. I will always feed you well and take good care of you. I will send my helicopter for you and all you have to do is come and 'be good to me'." All I wanted to do when he said that was to throw up and get the heck out of there. I didn't think it was a good idea to tell him that he grossed me out, so when I could, I politely got off his lap where he was holding me, and headed for the bathroom to think. After all, that is where any self-respecting girl would go when in trouble. I planned how to sneak out without him seeing me, and get the pilot to take me back to the 12th.

I left the bathroom, watching to be sure he couldn't see me go then looked for the pilot. When I found the pilot and told him that I wanted to go back to the 12th Evac Hospital he said, "No way. Not until tomorrow."

I told him, "I am not staying here with these guys until tomorrow" and went to walk around. The audacity of the officers to assume we would stay the night with them! So here I was in a foreign country, in the middle of a war, at a strange hospital far from my home base. Since it was a hospital, I decided to walk around and see if I could find a nurse to help me. As I walked, I heard a male voice from between two buildings, and became wary. He saw my body react and said, "It's Okay, Ma'am, I am friendly."

I answered, "How do I know that?"

He came out into the light where I could see him, and I saw he was like so many other nineteen-year-olds I had seen at the 12th, and he was enlisted. That meant he was likely to treat me more respectfully. The officers had the attitude, as did the general, that I was government property. It would take much more than an act of Congress to make a gentleman out of many of those guys. The enlisted men were just glad to be able to talk and share. I told the young man my predicament and he said that I could sleep on one of the wards that night, and go back on the chopper in the morning. So that is what I did.

What a night that was. I was tense and unsure all night, listening to the wounded soldiers moan and cry; I did not sleep much. I do remember doing a lot of praying that night, that I would be safe while I slept and I was. Because I was an OR nurse, I had no idea what it was like on a ward until that night. The next day, I went back to the 12th and told my chief nurse, "If that is an example of the parties I get invited to, I would rather not go. I will stay here and work instead."

That didn't mean I didn't do things for fun, I did. I went to dances at the officers' club and I drank Mai Tai's, or rum and Coke and danced for hours. Dancing was how I got out my feelings. It was like the dance of the tarantella, intense, to get all the toxins out. Sometimes, at the clubs I would talk about the casualties that got to me emotionally. The guys that heard me couldn't take it, and so they would add liquor to my drinks. The more I drank, the more I talked and the more graphic I became. I was pretty vulnerable then, and I was lucky that I was with guys who treated me with respect. Being an officer, I was not supposed to "fraternize with the enlisted," but they seemed to be the only ones that respected me and that I could talk with about life. I could talk for hours to a young guy from Florida who had red hair and freckles. I don't know what it was about the red headed guys there, but they seemed to be the ones I was drawn to and who were open and sensitive. We talked about our experiences, our feelings, our ideas, back home, our lives before the war, our dreams, etc.

We had cookouts whenever we could for whatever occasion there was. The food came from the mess sergeants and they set up a big barbecue in barrels cut in half lengthwise. The doctors and the sergeants would do the cooking and we could wear our civilian clothes during cookouts. Those times allowed us to be with each other and laugh, play, socialize, and eat well. This could go on as long as no helicopters came in. We did this even when choppers came in, but we stopped to watch, and sometimes when I was on call, I would leave to go to the OR. The cookouts were only about fifty yards from our helipad.

Volleyball was one of the forms of recreation we had. It was the most cutthroat volleyball I had ever seen. The men, doctors, officers, male nurses and technicians used that as their way of releasing their feelings and aggressions. They would hammer the ball, jump on one another, use obscenities, smash the ball with rage and knock each other over. None of the female nurses would join in after having one experience or seeing them, it was too risky. They played to kill.

We watched movies outside on a screen that was made of big white paper attached to a wooden frame. It was like what a mobile blackboard would look like only this one was white. The movies were usually old and not very good. If there was fighting nearby or helicopters coming in, it was very distracting. The movie area was the same area used for the volleyball court.

In the U.S. people take coffee or cigarette breaks, in Vietnam we took war breaks; we went outside to watch the war, it was that close. The 12th Evacuation Hospital was in the heat of the battle on the edge of the Iron Triangle; I could watch the jets strafing the Hobo Woods. At night we sat on the water tower and watched the gunships, flares and tracer bullets coming from the gunships, which were only about one mile away. One day B-52s dropped bombs about five miles away; the ground shook and the supplies in the OR went bouncing off the shelves. Across the road from us was an artillery battery where they had 105 mm guns, and eight-inch Howitzers that would fire and shake up our supplies also. Our eye surgeon had the artillery battery moved after he came, because of the delicate surgery he did and the risks when the guns went off and shook the table with the patient on it.

The enemies were the VC and the North Vietnamese; although during my tour it was all VC who wore black pajamas and had booby traps and tunnels all over the area. Underneath Cu Chi, where the 12th Evac was stationed, were 200 miles of tunnels that went from Saigon to beyond Cu Chi. Outside the OR was our outhouse, and beside it was the opening to one of those tunnels. While I was there, they told me there were no VC in the tunnels. I never believed them. How else did the VC always seem to know what we were doing and know when to hit us? I felt scared every time I had to use the outhouse by the OR. For one thing the mamma-san, Vietnamese women who worked on the basecamp, would use that toilet, and they stood on the toilet seat to relieve themselves, so the seat was always disgusting. And then, there was that tunnel opening — what if they came out of the opening and booby-trapped the bathroom? I always lived in fear that either I'd get blown up opening the door, or when I bent over to pee. I didn't want to be blown up, but most certainly not from my bottom. Whenever we had blood from our suction machines to dump, I would dump it down the tunnel opening and yell obscenities down the hole, with my anger, "You sneaky VC, why don't you come out and fight us face to face. Here is some American blood shed for your people and your country!" I hated that war and what it did to the beautiful country of Vietnam, and to so many people on both sides. I saw the beauty of the beaches there and the lush green vegetation, and then the ugly OD war machinery and weapons, or the gravel and torn up land. Side by side they showed the dreadful contrasts.

The VC used Punji[16] Sticks, Bouncing Betties[17] Claymore Mines[18], Satchel Charges, grenades, mortars, rockets, AK 47s and snipers to wipe out our personnel. To kill or capture an American nurse was very desirable to their cause and destructive to the morale of the Americans.

---

[16] Bamboo sticks that were sharpened and then rubbed with cow dung or water buffalo dung, then set in the ground in the jungle with the point sticking up so soldiers would get cut by it and get infected

[17] Bouncing betties were landmines that were set in the ground so that a soldier would trip it off and get blown up. They had metal shrapnel in them, or little pellets, that would be driven into the soldier's tissues.

[18] A fragmentation mine filled with metal balls that fan out and embed into ground troops bodies.

When a soldier was hit with a Bouncing Betty or Claymore Mine, we cut out each piece of shrapnel and cleaned all the wounds. After three days of having their bandages soaked and changed every four hours on the wards and receiving antibiotics, they returned to the OR for a Delayed Primary Closure (DPC). That is how we handled war wounds. They could not be closed right away, or they would become infected, which would lead to gas gangrene[19] and the patient's death. All war wounds were considered "dirty" and left open and cleansed over and over with normal saline for three days before being closed up.

I worked twelve to twenty hours a day doing surgery and cleaning up. Some soldiers came in after stepping on landmines and had their intestines full of shrapnel. There are five feet of large intestines in the human body, and we had to examine each and every inch of that, feeling along in six-to-eight-inch increments to make sure it was clear of shrapnel. Even then the surgeon would take that piece and roll it several times, a sort of double check, as even the tiniest piece of metal left behind could cause peritonitis[20] and death. If there was metal in it then he had to pick it out with forceps and sometimes he had to sew up the cut made by the metal. Once that section was clear we'd move on and do the next six inches in the same way, until we had run the whole bowel.

Eye surgery was tedious because the instruments were hard to see. The tips distinguished one from another and they were very tiny. Each instrument with a different tip had a name and some numbers also. I looked very carefully at each tip to know which instrument it was and to give the correct one to the surgeon when he asked for it. Our eye surgeon, Dr. Roland Houle, liked to work with me, as the other nurses did not like those tiny instruments, so whenever there was an eye case, they called me. I remember a soldier with a head wound who came to

---

[19] Gas gangrene is a fast-spreading and potentially life-threatening form of gangrene caused by a bacterial infection to traumatized muscle. The infection causes toxins to release gas, which leads to muscle death.

[20] Inflammation of the peritoneum the membrane that lines the abdominal cavity.

us from the 24th Evacuation Hospital where they did neurosurgery. The neurosurgeon at the 24th Evac examined the soldier and realized that if his eye was not taken care of first, the young man would lose his vision. They sent him to us on a dust-off and we did the eye surgery. The dust-offs had a red cross painted on the side to identify it as carrying wounded. According to the rules of the Geneva Convention, that meant the enemy should not fire at it. The VC and the North Vietnamese did not adhere to the rules of the Geneva Convention and they also knew if they could shoot down a dust-off or bomb a hospital, that it would have a negative effect on the morale of the U.S. troops so they used the red crosses for target practice.

We put this young soldier with the head and eye wound on our table. Dr. Houle examined him and said that we would need to repair the eye socket and put in an implant. The Silastic implant he used was a small triangle of white silicone material. The surgeon used wire to pull some of the bone together and to hold the implant in place after he seated it in the cracked eye socket. Roland was one of the nicest doctors there; he took his life and his work seriously and didn't drink alcohol or fool around with nurses, like the other docs did.

In Vietnam there were two seasons, hot and wet and hot and dry. During the hot and dry season, the land was brown, the sun miserably hot, the air so dry it would suck the moisture from the land. When the wind blew it would stir up the dirt which would get into everything when we opened the door. As the season went along, the sky itself would be filled, turning it brown and filling the air with the smell of dirt, dust, metal, fire powder, and, more than anything else, war. Sometimes at the hospital, the wind blew the brown dirt around so much that I could hardly see 100 yards in front of me.

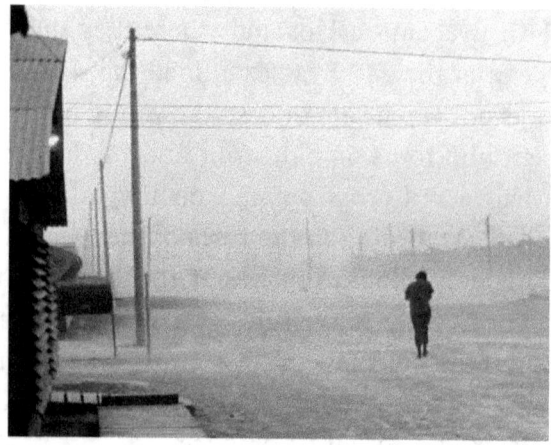
11. My friend, Connie Jean Evans, walking during a chinook. (winds)

During the hot and wet season, the land was lush and green like Washington State, and the air smelled tropical and fresh, except for the nasty war smells; or it was muggy hot, with a heavier more intense flavor to the smells. Several times during hot and wet monsoon season, I had to stand in four to six inches of water while doing surgery. When the artillery went off across the road, some of our sterile supplies would jump around on the shelves and fall on the cement floor into the rainwater. When that happened, we had to take the cover off, wash it and re-sterilize the whole package. Our sterilizers were big round tanks of OD metal that built up steam and pressure inside for long enough to kill any bacteria in the items we were sterilizing. Our sterilizers were so old they looked like they were from WWII.

Mortar attacks could come at any time, and when they did, it was terrifying. I always knew it could be the one that leaves me wounded or killed. I felt it deep in my gut each time. The most terrifying were while I was scrubbed in on a case, and once while I was in a jeep. I had never performed surgery during an attack before and when this attack started, I suddenly realized that now we would have to use the protocol that I learned in basic training; that the surgeon is the highest-ranking officer and he would decide what each person would do and when.

On this day when the attack started, I was scrubbed in with the chief of surgery, who was a major. He looked at me and said, "You and I will work fast and finish this case." He turned to the anesthetist, a male nurse, and said, "You get under the table and keep working; if she and I get hit, you finish the surgery and then get help."

The anesthetist and the corpsman took cover under the steel OR table, the patient was wide open, while the surgeon and I finished sewing up the bowel and then closed the abdomen. As the mortars were whistling in, I remember instinctively ducking my head, even though that would do me no good at all if one of them hit. We did not have sandbag cover over the OR, so if a mortar hit us, we'd all be dead. We had only a thin sheet of metal between the mortar round and us, if it hit the OR. My hand shook as I threaded the needles one handed with 4-0 black silk. I could not use my other hand to steady it because it was busy holding an abdominal retractor so that the surgeon could see into the abdomen. I worked as fast as I could to keep up, feeling scared that I would die, and mad that I was so vulnerable standing there with mortars aimed right at us. The combination of feelings and mortars coming in didn't help me act with any finesse, but we did get it done. I was clumsier than usual with my hand shaking. When we were done, we put the patient under the table for cover and I went down there with him. The attack ended shortly after that, and fortunately there was no damage to the hospital or injury to any of our people; but we did end up with a lot of casualties from around the base-camp. Thank God, their aim with the mortars was not very accurate. We were one of their main targets.

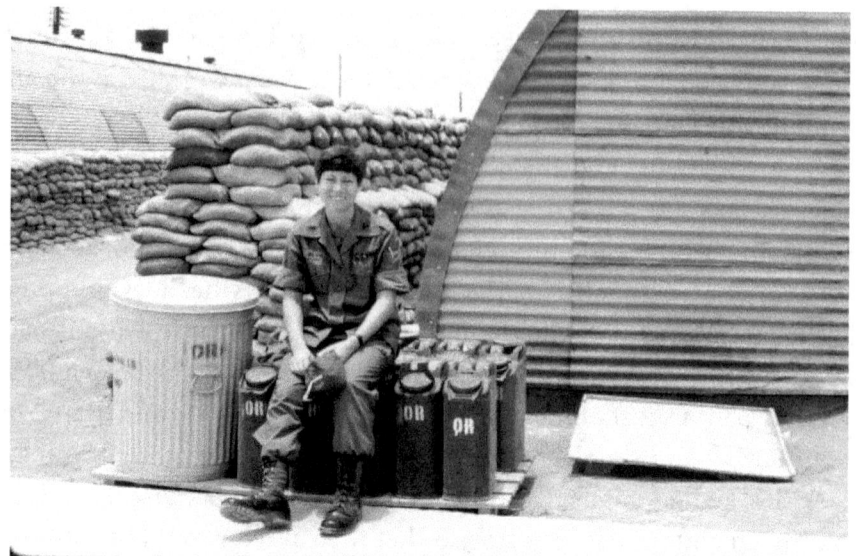

12. Me sitting on water cans with sandbags visible. Those were to protect us but since they only went up about four feet they would not help if a mortar round hit us even if it hit exactly between the rows of sand bags.

The other worst incident with a mortar attack came when I was with an officer in a jeep trying to get back to the hospital quickly because of the attack. The jeep was wide open and I felt like a sitting duck. He drove wildly to get me back to the hospital and him back to his unit.

Another enemy we had to deal with were the locusts. They were reddish brown in color about two inches long, and would hop and fly. These locusts came about twice a year in the thousands and swarmed all over. They flew into the OR when the door was opened for someone to come or go and they landed right in or on open wounds. We called them nurse killers and when we killed them, we put a large gauge needle through them and put them on our bulletin boards. At our hooch, they usually swarmed in the outhouses so we went there two at a time — one nurse could bat them away with a broom, while the other nurse did what she needed to do there.

Our hospital was across the road to our south from the petroleum dump, and across the western road from the artillery battery. It was also down the eastern road from the helicopters, and not far from the

Military Area Radio Station (MARS). Each of those was a major military target. I never understood why they put the hospital in such a vulnerable spot on the base camp, and well understood my drill sergeant's reaction when he learned I was being stationed at the 12th Evacuation Hospital. The MARS was where we got to call home, maybe twice a year, if we were lucky. The call would go to a radio ham operator who would relay it to another ham operator until they got close enough to our home state to make the call. It was different than talking on the phone, and of course there was no privacy at all; all the guys at the MARS and all the radio operators along the way could hear everything.

I did make at least two calls home on that system. It sounded like this: "Hi Mom, Dad. How is everything at home? Any news for me? Over." They would share what they could of the local news and how they were doing and would ask me how I was doing. "Over" Saying over let the ham radio operator know to switch to me as speaker. "We are as busy as ever with mass casualties coming in several times a week. Dad, we have an eye surgeon who could use some of your jeweler's forceps to remove shrapnel from eyes. Can you send me some? We can autoclave them so he could use them in surgery. Mom, please send some salt water taffy and the taffy paddles for me and the other nurses?"

# Chapter 3
# UP CLOSE AND PERSONAL IN VIETNAM – PART 2

October 18th, 1967, when the Manchus were hit, (4th Battalion 9th Regiment of the 25th Infantry Division.) was a day like many others except that I have memory of one specific guy and his hand. We had already done a full day's work when Jim showed up. I was tired both physically and emotionally and had been numb for many months. Jim grabbed my hand in his bloody one, looked into my eyes, pleading with me. His eyes and his voice were full of intensity when he said to me: "I am a baseball pitcher — you've gotta save my hand!" Jim had wounds all over his body, as so many did. I knew his hand was not our priority, but it certainly was his. Our surgical team went to work on his belly wounds and leg wounds and after about three hours all his wounds except the hand were taken care of. As I was preparing his hand for the surgeon to work on it, the surgeon, who was the chief of surgery, leaned over to me and said, "I am going next door to work on another case, you take care of his hand."

"But sir," I said, "He is a baseball pitcher and I am not even a surgeon. I can't do that! I need YOU to sew it up!" The surgeon shook his head and I implored, "Sir, he really needs a surgeon to sew up his hand, not a nurse!" The surgeon was already moving next door while I was imploring him not to have me sew up Jim's hand.

My corpsman was looking at me, the nurse anesthetist was looking at me — and I was looking at Jim's hand. The heat of Vietnam and the stench of war penetrated and filled the Quonset hut, and what rose up in me was rage. *How can I be expected to do what a surgeon trains for years to do? What if I ruin his hand? I felt like I could kill anyone or anything right then. Oh shit! what am I going to do?*

"Okay," I said to my corpsman, "let's prep his hand and get me the finest silk suture material we have." I took in some deep breaths, and, had it been somewhere between January and March, probably would have said a prayer, but I'd lost my faith completely by then, so it was going to be just me doing this.

My corpsman washed Jim's hand with Betadine and covered his arm, and the board it was resting on, with sterile cloth. He brought me a chair to sit on while I looked at Jim's mutilated hand. And then, without even realizing it, I began to pray, probably something from my years of habit. In that moment, wanting to do my best for this soldier, this baseball player, I forgot my anger at God, my resentment of him for turning a blind eye to all of this devastation. *I am not an artist or a surgeon, how in the world can I do a good job for this guy?* I wanted to cry — but that was out of the question and not even possible since I had long ago locked up anything resembling grief or sadness. It was too risky here to have those feelings. I learned within days of coming here that what showed on my face was read by the soldiers to mean the worst for them. If I looked sad or started to cry, they immediately believed it meant they were going to die. All of my feelings had to be locked up — and they were.

I began to pick up edges of skin on each side of Jim's palm and gently approximate it to the other side to see how far it could go. Gradually I was starting to see how the sides of the wound could possibly come together, but also knew and felt in my gut, that no matter what I did or how I did it, Jim was likely going to have a thick scar right down through the palm of his pitching hand because, *dammit, I am not a hand surgeon! I am not even a surgeon! I am just an OR nurse and I* should not be the one doing this! OK, I told myself, quit it, that will not help. Breathe...Focus and do the best you can.

I threaded a small curved needle with the blue 6.0 silk and took a deep breath as I pushed the needle through the edge of the loose skin and began to gently pull it over to the most likely place on the other side of the wound so it would lay flat. *Do I do one at a time or connect them all? What do I remember seeing? Some of each, I think.* I tied the first one off so it would stay where it was and I could take one at a time. The next one was close to the first one and I tied that one off too. Then someone opened the door and in flew a swarm of locusts. *OH NO!* It looked like about twenty-thirty came through the door. I could see and hear all the corpsman going after them. I had to stay focused on what I was doing but then one of the locusts landed right on Jim's wound. "Get that damned thing off there right now or I am out of here!" My corpsman, Howie, was a good guy that I liked working with and he knew I meant what I said, so he was beside me instantly. The trick was to get the locust out while maintaining the sterility. "Use a sterile glove, Howie." I could see the light dawning on him and he opened up some sterile gloves, put one on and used the other to move the locust out of the way. Within minutes, the locusts were pinned to the corkboard skewered with a needle, our kill for the day.

With no air conditioning the inside temperature was about 115 degrees, and it was 105 outside. The sweat was pouring off my face and about to go into the wound, so Howie came over and I turned away from Jim to let Howie wipe the sweat from my eyes and face. Back to Jim's hand — one stitch at a time. It was like putting a puzzle together, but he was a pitcher and needed to be able to feel with this hand to control the baseball. There was a small area where I felt like I could put several stitches together without tying each one off. My fingers were not adept at tying this fine silk suture material and I felt clumsy. After all, *I AM NOT A SURGEON!* My mind screamed my anger and rage at being in this position.

Okay... back to the task at hand. One more stitch and it looked like it was all closed. "Whew! So glad that's done. I am so afraid he is not going to be happy with this after it heals and it won't work for him the way he wants." I said that out loud to no one or anyone who could hear.

Then I washed and washed his hand wound and put a wad of Kerlix (prewashed, fluff-dried 100% woven gauze in a crinkle-weave pattern to cushion and protect) in his palm before I wrapped it up. I knew the nurses on the wards would remove the bandages every four hours and irrigate the wound before they rebandaged it. The Kerlix (would hopefully prevent the hand and fingers from contracting too much.

Then it was on to the next wounded soldier. Another Manchu. *How many more today?* That day we had many more after Jim. The Manchus had never been hit that badly before. I knew their lieutenant was going to have a lot to deal with after all that. So many of them were badly wounded and I never knew what happened to them. In the case of Jim Vines, I did later learn he did some pitching when he got back but not as well as he would have liked and it was too hard to continue. He told me in 2014, that the most important part to him was that he used that hand to put the wedding ring on his wife's finger.

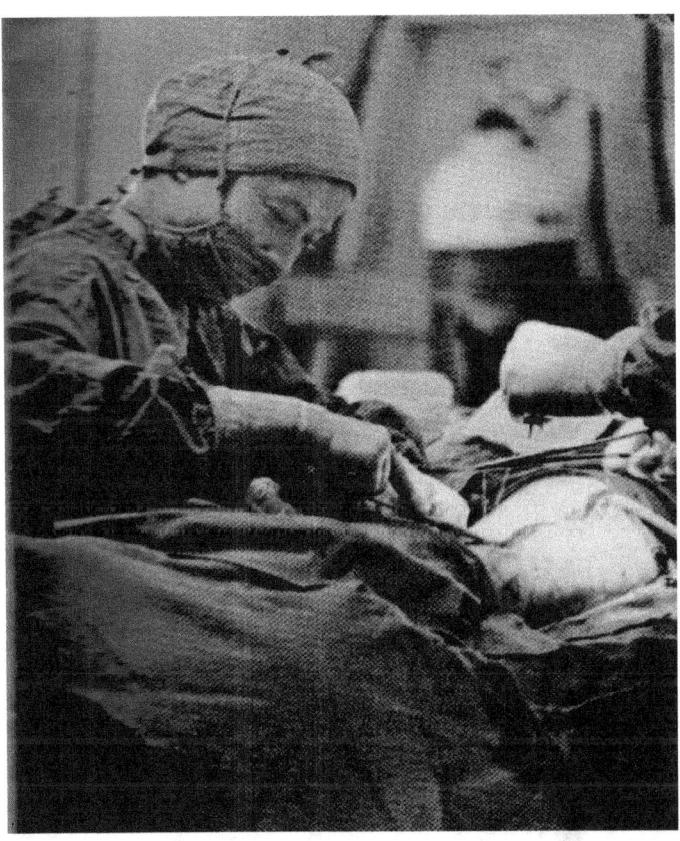

13. Closing up a soldier's abdomen. Photo by Raymond Cranbourne-Empire/"Angels of Viet Nam," Today's Health, August 1967.

Vietnam was a beautiful country, very green, with truly sweet people. The Vietnam War replaced the beauty with ugliness, and the sweetness with bitterness. A once beautiful country was decimated by our war there. Making it even worse was the vicious cycle our young soldiers seemed to be stuck in. They would be sent out to secure an area, such as a camp located on the exquisitely green Nui Ba Dinh, the Black Virgin Mountain in Tay Ninh, taking it after a hard-fought battle. But then, only a week later, lose it back to the Viet Cong (VC).

We had units on top of the mountain and at the bottom while the VC had units in the middle. The two sides constantly exchanged holdings, fighting again and again to take the same area. It made no sense to me or to some of our soldiers. If the U.S. won a small piece of land, what would we do with it? It was infuriating for me and devastating for our soldiers when their units were ambushed or caught in crossfire after being called to help an ARVN unit (Army of the Republic of Vietnam, South Vietnamese soldiers). I learned quickly there was no trust between our guys and theirs, and there were weekly stories of our soldiers being set up by the ARVNs, where many of our men were killed and permanently injured. I knew within my first two weeks that this war was all wrong and so many of my experiences supported that. Nothing I went through during the war or afterwards ever changed that belief.

During the first six months of my tour, I clung to my faith in God and went to the chapel on post when I could. A few times I was able to sneak out of base camp to attend the Catholic Church in Cu Chi. The priest was Father Fond and the Mass was either in Latin or Vietnamese. Though whenever I went, I always prayed for my safety, as well as for those around me, more so I would pray for the war to end and the horror to stop.

I was never really safe, and the war went on and on, continuing for many more years even after I returned home. Yet it wasn't until Johnny came in and I "snapped" that I lost my faith in God. I could not believe that the God of Love that I knew could allow such atrocities to take place daily — and for the utter destruction of the beautiful land of Vietnam and so many people, both Americans and Vietnamese. I think I disconnected from God but my faith was so long held from childhood I am sure I wavered back and forth. I was not the same after the day Johnny came in. All of my memories of Vietnam are in color until that day, and from then on, they are all black and white or sepia toned. I think I became more cynical for those last six months and I drank a lot more than my first six months; I did not believe I would live to see home again.

We had many different kinds of cases, like a bleeder to find and tie off, or a circumcision. We did a lot of circumcisions over there because of the heat and dirt that the guys had to endure, and their sexual activities with the Vietnamese women. They were very painful operations to have in those circumstances and the guys were always very embarrassed when a female nurse was scrubbed in for a circumcision. Another kind of case was to reopen a wound such as a chest wound, where something was going on inside that the surgeon needed to see and correct.

Supplies were a big problem for us; we ran out of many things we really needed all the time, like catgut suture, lap sponges used in abdominal cases to soak up the blood in the belly, and razor blades used to shave off hair. Even in stateside surgeries patients were shaved all around the surgical wound to have the cleanest area possible. We had to do a lot of shaving; sometimes whole bodies, so we constantly ran out of the straight razors.

We also often did not have the tiny stainless-steel forceps used to take shrapnel out of eyes and we ran out of surgical light bulbs to operate by. It was very frustrating. We were doing our best to help the soldiers and were thwarted by the people who sent us there.

I learned very early, that if we needed something, I had to do something to get it. I knew nurses at other hospitals and called to tell them what we needed and they did the same. We each looked for what we had that was extra, or an excess of, to barter or exchange. I would have to fly on the chopper to their hospital to do the exchange, because no one ever wanted to come to Cu Chi, it was too dangerous. An aunt of mine owned a grocery store and mailed me boxes of straight razor blades so we could continue to prepare the soldiers appropriately for surgery. My dad, who was a jeweler, sent me three pair of small jeweler tweezers I had seen in his store that were stainless steel and could be sterilized. We used those tweezers as forceps and saved the eyesight of many a young GI who had shrapnel removed from their eyes with them. For the lap sponges (large white soft material about eight-by-eight inches) we had to improvise and use towels instead. What I couldn't barter for, we went without.

In the first six months, I met a young air force pilot who flew the single engine bird dog planes that marked areas for the jets to strafe. He and I became good friends and liked to dance together at his officers' club. It was a small club and some of my nurse friends were dating guys in the same officers' club. There were about six of us who hung out together. I drank rum and Coke or a Mai Tai and tried to work out my emotions by dancing wildly. There were a few times when the other guys would double up on the alcohol in my drink to get me to talk more. I would usually spout off about the horrible things I saw and felt from the cases we had that day. The more I said and the uglier it sounded, the worse it was for them — and they would stop me from drinking.

There were various politicians and celebrities that would come over to get publicity. Rarely did we see any who came because they cared. Martha Raye was one who cared and so was Charlton Heston. For some reason we knew ahead of time when Charlton Heston was coming. I informed our chief of surgery that I planned to see Charlton Heston when he arrived and told him the timing. I asked him NOT to schedule anything during that time. On the day Charlton Heston was to arrive, our chief of surgery did schedule a case at the very time I asked him not to. I told him I would not scrub in for it but my corpsman would. The sergeant on the post-op ward notified me when Charlton Heston was there and I left to see him. On a note pad he took down the names and phone numbers of soldier's families and called them when he returned home.

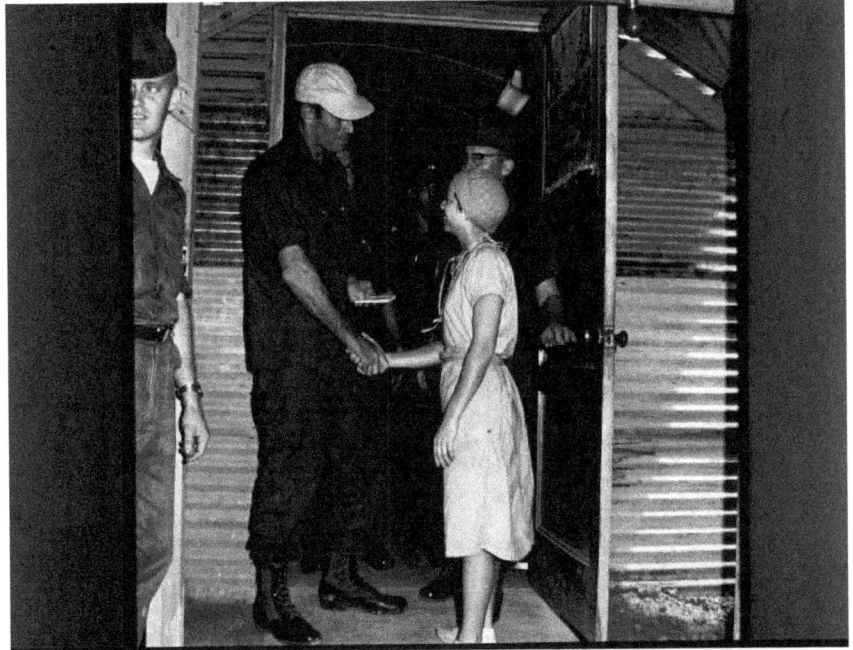

14. My meeting with Charlton Heston the actor who played the role of Moses in the movie The Ten Commandments.

• • • • •

Here was a typical day for me in Vietnam.

I woke up at 5:30 am, went to the latrine to pee, and then took a cold shower. I washed fast and woke up immediately from the cold water. I climbed into my fatigues and boots, checked my bed for creatures and insects then remade my bed with the green OR sheets that I washed myself. On top of the sheets was my OD nylon poncho liner, which I dearly loved and kept me warm at night. I tucked in my mosquito netting as tight as I could under my mattress, the tighter the better to keep the rats off. They ran along the two x fours at night. The two x fours were located about twelve inches above my head along the length of the bed and beyond. As I made my bed, I heard the sounds of the other nurses in the hooch moaning and groaning, some talking about the worst case the night before, and some listening to armed forces radio. I found my baseball cap and reluctantly put it on to walk to the mess hall. It was protocol to have a head covering so we had to wear those ugly OD baseball caps when we were outside buildings. I stopped for my buddy Claire, and we walked together to the mess hall.

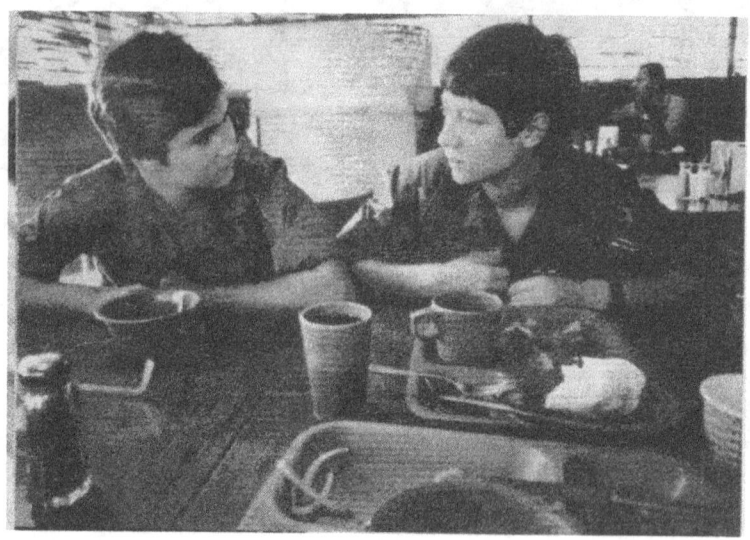

15. In the mess hall with my buddy Claire. Photo by Raymond Cranbourne-Empire/Angels of Viet Nam Today's Health, August 1967.

As we passed the other hooches and the hospital Quonset huts, we saw a soldier in his blue army issue pajamas smoking outside the door. The mess hall trucks were delivering breakfast to the wards, and we heard the sounds of the nurses working on patients inside. It was Monday, so we couldn't go into the mess hall until we took our malaria pills. We swallowed them and went in to get breakfast. I told the soldier serving that I wanted six eggs over easy and he told me for the 100th time, you can only have two. I tell him (for the 100th time) that I am an OR nurse, and I will be doing surgery on his buddies all morning with no breaks, and I need six eggs to get me through. He looked behind him and got a nod from the NCO, and I got my six eggs. I loaded up with toast and juice and went to the table where Claire was already sitting. I stepped over the bench to get in and sat down. Our tables were like picnic tables. The benches were straight and long, held about six of us, and were connected to the table, so we had to lift our legs and step over to get in. We ate in silence for a while and then one of the surgeons sat with us. He was loud and sarcastic and his voice filled the air. He was angry and resentful and he let everyone know that.

One of the other surgeons came to the table with tears in his eyes said: "I am dreading one of the cases I have today. It is a DPC on a guy who lost his legs, one arm and one eye. I don't know how that guy will want to live that way. I hate this war and what it is doing!"

We finished breakfast and Claire and I headed over to the OR. Once there, we changed into our scrubs (a green OR dress and hair cap, and blood-stained sneakers that used to be light green). We both checked the schedule to see which cases were coming and what supplies we would need. We got the supplies and put them in the areas with the OR tables. I went to the scrub sink as soon as my tech came to open the packs. The patient was brought in and I talked with him briefly until the nurse anesthetist put him to sleep. He told me, "I'm from Florida and glad that I can go home after this surgery. I sure hope my girlfriend won't be freaked out by my wounds and scars." In my heart I believed she probably would be freaked out. The tech went over to the patient and helped to put his arm on the board for the intravenous (IV) where the fluids and some anesthesia began going into his veins during the case. Then the tech scrubbed all the skin around the wounds for twenty minutes each.

The surgeon came in scrubbed, and I put the gown on him and held the gloves while he plunged his hands down deep into each glove. The glove stretched and came halfway up his arm then receded back down to about four inches above his wrist. Finally, the tech tied the back of the surgeon's gown. The surgeon looked at the nurse anesthetist and waited for the nod to go ahead with the case.

We did the case, a DPC. The edges of each wound were brought together and sewn up. Catgut was used to sew the muscle and fascia, and silk to sew up the skin. Once the wounds were all closed, we put on clean bandages and sent the patient back to recovery, and then we cleaned up. Clean up meant all the sheets were put in a laundry hamper, all the instruments went in the large steel basin and on to central supply, then we washed down the tables with alcohol and scrubbed the cement floor with a wet mop.

Once all that was done, I changed my gown and gloves. I kept them on during clean up so I did not have to do another twenty-minute scrub of my hands and arms. I would simply strip off the previous gown and gloves, without touching my skin to anything, and then put on a new sterile gown and set of sterile gloves. The gloves were packed so they have a cuff with the inside turned out. I could touch the inside of the cuff to get the glove on and then using that sterile glove go under the cuff to touch the sterile part of the second glove and put it on the other hand. Once the sterile glove is on the second hand, I completed the gloving of the first hand, touching only the sterile part. We then set up the sheets, doctor's gown and gloves and all the instruments, the suture material, basin with syringe and the saline for the next case.

We continued doing DPCs the rest of the day and probably went through about six in my area. Multiply that by five room areas going all day. At the end of the day, at about four pm, I went over to central supply and helped with the cleaning and packing of instruments, instrument trays, plus the cleaning and powdering of gloves. We reused any gloves that did not have holes in them. We washed them and put water in them to check for holes, then dried them outside on a clothesline.

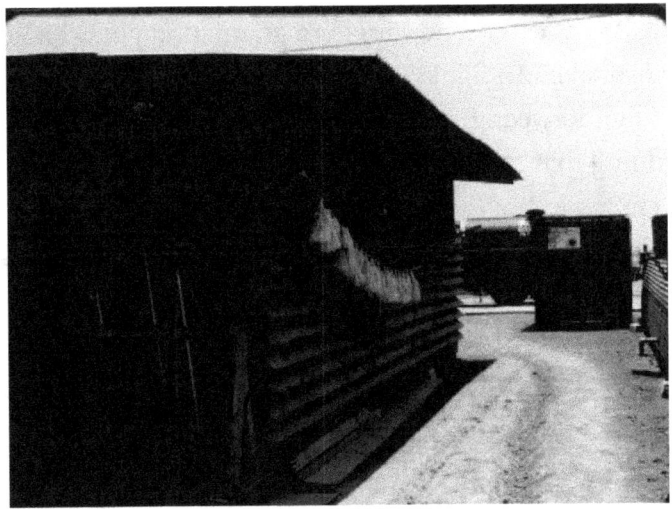

16. Gloves drying outside of central supply.
Water truck in background

Finally, we powdered them, put them into the green cloth cases, one glove on each side, then wrapped the case in a green square of material, taped it shut and sterilized them.

When that was all completed, we went to the mess hall for dinner. For lunch during the day, we rotated out to the mess hall or the lunch crew brought sandwiches over to us. It was not uncommon for me to eat between cases with my scrub gown and gloves on. I simply washed my gloved hands and ate and then switched again.

Dinner was meatloaf and mashed potatoes with peas and carrots and some canned fruit for dessert, along with the usual iced tea or Kool-Aid to drink. I hate Kool-Aid so drank iced tea with a lot of lemon and sugar. The tea was very bitter without it. I looked around for a place to sit. Claire was with Jim, her anesthesiologist boyfriend, so I joined my head nurse, Liz, and a couple other nurses who worked on the wards. We talked about the day. Someone had news from the U.S. and shared it, while everyone listened. The news was about baseball and other summer activities. That started a discussion of home and what we were missing. One of the nurse's brothers would be graduating from high school and she was sad that she will not be there. He lettered in gymnastics and will be getting some awards and she will be missing it.

She asked, "What can I send him for a graduation gift?" Liz's friend in another hospital had a fight with her chief nurse over the mamma sans stealing her underwear. Liz is laughing as she tells the story, because her friend is doing that to keep the chief nurse occupied while they play a joke on her.

After dinner I went to the hooch and wondered how long I could be there before something happened and I was called back to the OR. At the hooch I talked with some of my hooch mates, loud classical music was playing, someone was singing, and we stopped talking to listen. Maybe forty-five minutes went by when we heard the first chopper came in. I was on call so ran over to the OR and got into my scrubs. I asked my corpsman to check pre-op to see how many cases came in, and what they were. What they are meant, belly or chest wounds, all over body wounds, amputations, etc. He came back and told me only four casualties came in and they didn't look too bad. He said to set up for two cases. We set it up and he called over to the hooch for another nurse. As we were setting up, we heard another chopper. My corpsman looked out the door and told me they were off loading another six casualties, and these looked worse than the first few he saw. Liz came in then and said we would be working four tables. She called Claire back; Liz and Claire both scrubbed as several corpsman arrived.

We each scrubbed for the mandatory twenty minutes with Betadine from fingertips to elbows, then I went to my assigned area to put on a sterile gown and gloves. My tech tied my gown in the back and I prepared the stainless-steel basin and the bulb syringe. My corpsman poured the sterile saline into the basin that we would use to wash out the wounds. The bulb syringe was large and had a large red rubber ball at the end that fit into my gloved hand. I squeezed it to draw up the saline into the glass tube and later would squeeze it into the wound to send in the saline solution.

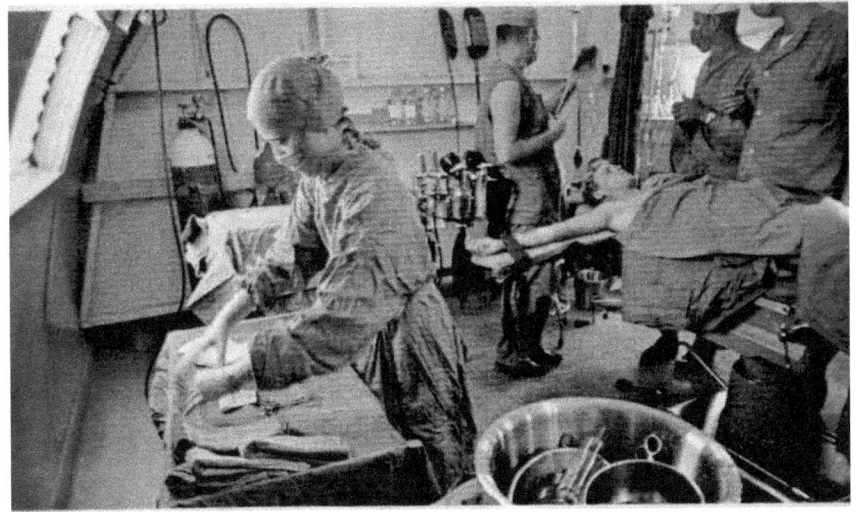

17. Soldier on OR table, the anesthetist, 2 technicians and me at the back table. Note stainless steel basin and bulb syringe. Photo by Raymond Cranbourne-Empire/"Angels of Viet Nam," Today's Health, August 1967.

Next, I would set up the sterile sheets so that I knew where each one was and could use it when needed. The sheets were used to drape over the patient, and the one with the large hole went over the surgical opening. I put the doctor's sterile gown and gloves close to the edge of the table so I could get to them easily when the surgeon was scrubbed in. Next, I would set up all the instruments on the Mayo stand, which sat over the patient and put some instruments on my back table. I needed to know every instrument and where it was. Next, I told my tech what sutures would be needed for the case and he opened each suture packet.

We were set up for the first case and the soldier came in. I saw that he was losing a lot of blood and had both a leg and a belly wound. The chief of surgery arrived and said to get started while he scrubbed. I called for an abdominal instrument pack and added it to what I already had on the back table. I had three packs of catgut rolled up on rubber tubing and set up the instruments that I thought we would use on the Mayo stand. I knew the abdominal retractor this surgeon liked and asked my corpsman to have it handy to open. I checked the scissors and made sure they were working well, because this surgeon is very picky about that. The chief of surgery re-entered as the patient was going under the anesthetic. The tech was still scrubbing the skin around the wounds as I gowned and gloved the surgeon and started handing him sheets. On this case we used the sheet with the hole in it to go over the belly wound. When my corpsman was finished, he went behind the surgeon and tied his gown.

We were ready to start and the surgeon went for the bleeders first. I handed him the hemostats he asked for and he tied off the bleeders. He then started to explore to see what was in the wound. He carefully checked around inside and found no metal. An AK 47 hit this young man and the round went right through from front to back. The surgeon said, "What a lucky hit for him, nothing major was damaged. Amazing! This guy must have had someone watching over him. It is a million-dollar wound because it will get him home early with minimal damage." After he explored the front wound and we washed it out, we turned the patient up on his side to scrub and check out the back wound. The major told us we couldn't leave these open and that he would put in a Penrose drain (a paper-thin piece of rubber tubing about ¾" wide and four-six" long) and he used catgut and wire to close the abdominal wound. We washed the patient's abdominal cavity with three bottles of saline and began the closure. After we finished with the abdominal wound, the surgeon went to pre-op in his gown and gloves, while we prepped the patient's leg wound and cleared off the abdominal instruments. When the surgeon came back he told us who was next. We completed the leg wound, cleaned up quickly and set up for the next case.

The next case was a big guy who was bleeding profusely from a lacerated liver. Livers are very deep dark red colored organs, soft and smooth to the touch; they detoxify impurities in the body and are rich in blood, so when cut, they bleed out excessively. No one can survive without a liver, so when we were faced with lacerated livers from firepower of some type, the surgeon cut out the wounded part and sewed up the edges. We used heavy catgut on a very large curved thick needle called a liver needle which is curved like a half moon, has a point followed by a flat section, then the rest of the curve is rounded steel. This soldier had a large pressure bandage over his liver that was keeping him alive.

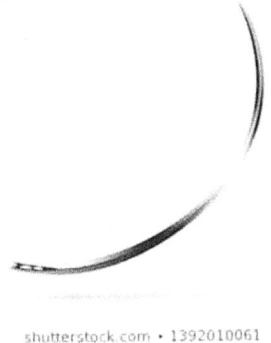

18. Liver needle.

We set up and did our best to keep the pressure on while we shaved the hair off around the wound and scrubbed the skin over his abdomen and chest. Luckily, he didn't have a lot of chest hair to shave. The corpsman had gotten the three retractors we were likely to use, so they were ready to open when the doctor asked for them. The surgeon kept on his sterile gown and gloves so he did not need to scrub again. He came in, looked at the patient and took off his contaminated gown and gloves and got into the new sterile set and saw the nod from the anesthetist. He put out his hand and said, "Scalpel." I slapped the scalpel into his hand and he made a long, angular, clean cut right through the laceration so that the surgical incision was longer and larger than the wound. He handed me the bloody scalpel as he asked for the large Metzenbaum scissors and cut quickly through the fascia and muscle to reveal the liver. He asked for an upper abdominal retractor, placed it under the ribcage and had me hold it firmly as he put both hands in the opening. He gently held the liver, looking for the laceration. The laceration he found was quite large and he wasn't sure he could sew it up. He continued to examine and considered his options as the clamps kept the bleeding to a minimum. Finally, he said that we were going to do a resection in order to have a clean area to suture. He cut away the part of the liver that had been injured and began to sew up the liver's edges with the large curved liver needle and heavy catgut.

I was being a surgeon with my left hand, holding the retractor and my right hand was threading the needles and handing them to him. He asked for a different retractor that worked mechanically to hold open the wound, so that both my hands were free to thread the needles and pass the instruments. I put the needle in a clamp and then slapped the clamp handle into the surgeon's hand. Holding the clamp, he angled it to slide into one liver edge and through to the other side using a right turning rotation of his wrist. We continued until the liver edges were completely sewn together with no visible bleeding or oozing around the sutures. When the surgeon was satisfied with the results, he did a complete exam inside the abdomen to be sure he has not missed anything before we closed up the wound.

We sewed the other tissues and the covering over the organs, then used wire for the skin and lastly, put in a drain. At the end of the case, the surgeon thanked all of us for our help and told us to take a fifteen-minute break before bringing in the next casualty. We cleaned up and got everything ready to go for the next case. My corpsman and I alternated taking our breaks, so we didn't lose valuable time. Sandwiches were brought in about two hours after the first chopper landed, so I grabbed one and some reconstituted powdered milk then headed to the break room next door after washing my gloved hands.

We had two surgery buildings; the second one had our dressing room and a small lounge area where we could take a break. I sat in the break room to eat and then went back to the other building to continue on with the next wounded soldier. I stripped off the sterile gown and gloves and put on a new set without touching anything, so that I did not have to do another twenty-minute scrub.

The next case was yet another young soldier who was losing the lower part of one leg hit by a grenade. We cleaned it up and took off the part that was attached by only a few strands of ligament and skin. We tied off the bleeders and cut out the dead muscle destroyed by the blast. When it was looking healthy, we washed it over and over with saline and then bandaged his stump. We checked to be sure there was no other metal in his body from the grenade, and then sent him to post-op.

While we were doing our cases, Claire and Liz were in the adjoining rooms doing theirs. After many hours and cases, it appeared that we might be done for the day. The surgeon came back to tell us that there were no new casualties and that we could clean up and go back to the hooch. We did that and just as we were heading out the door to go to the hooch, about 11:45 pm, we hear another chopper. Tired and ready to sleep, yet alert and prepared, we waited by pre-op to see what it was. The chopper set down, the pilot was yelling, and the guys with the stretcher run to the chopper but saw no casualties. The pilot was still yelling and the techs ran around to the other side and saw an officer in the front seat slumped over and bleeding. They got him on the stretcher and we finally heard some details. It turned out that the pilot was hit by gunfire from below. He took a hit right up into his armpit. The soldier yelling was not a pilot at all, but he did fly the chopper in. I could see by the pilot's arm that it required surgery, and since I was on call, I turned back to the OR and got into my scrubs again. As soon as I did, in came Major Stuart Poticha, the chief of surgery, who told me to set up for a vascular case.

After we got everything ready, they brought in the pilot who had a bloody wound that went from the top of his shoulder and around under his armpit. There were three clamps hanging out from under his arm where the bleeders were. We started prepping him and our supplies. I needed lots of silk suture material and some sterile mineral oil. I oiled the suture material that would be used to delicately approximate the edges of both sides of his brachial and axillary arteries, which were severed. The artery was slippery and difficult for the surgeon to sew and the case was tedious. The surgeon had to take the edges very carefully into his forceps, so as not to damage them, and then take very tiny stitches all the way around the artery, bringing the edges together evenly. For me, it was delicate as well because I had oil on my gloved fingers that I ran the silk through before passing it on to the surgeon. We were there into the early morning hours and finally, we were done again and this time I was hoping to get into my bed and sleep.

The early morning was quiet, and I felt hungry and exhausted as I got into my very cold shower, which woke me up. I cringed taking my late night/early morning cold showers, but always did it because I wanted to wash off the blood that splattered on me during surgery. I wanted the sight of it off me and especially the smell out of my head, even though the shower never succeeded in doing the latter.

Now I was even hungrier. After I was clean, I raided my stash of Beanie Weenies, a small can of cut up hotdogs and beans, which was a great quick snack to fill the hole before I could go to sleep. I ate, drank some water and listened to the sound of the other nurses sleeping. When I finished eating, I brushed my teeth and finally laid down in my bed and tucked in my mosquito netting and before I could think, I was sound asleep.

I woke up the next morning to the oppressive heat of the day and to the bright sun heating the side of the hooch. Another day of my life, gone. I was alive and the war went on. I smelled the shit pots burning. The excrement from the latrine pots had to be burned daily. Everyday about 9:30 a.m., a crew went around and removed all the pots and put clean ones in. They then set fire to the excrement. The black smoke curved and curled upward into our beautiful soft blue sky and not only made its visual mark on my senses, but the smell was uniquely pungent and unpleasant. Those shit pots were a major focus of the nurses because we often talked together about what we would do if we were ever overrun, i.e., if the enemy got through the perimeter and were on our base camp headed to the hospital. We were always told that our job was to protect the patients and get them to safety; guard the patients with our life. We believed that if we were overrun, none of our lives were safe and we would not be much good guarding the patients since we didn't have weapons. Our plan was to hide out in the shit pots. We even spoke about taking cyanide pills rather than be captured. Our guys, soldiers, technicians, and pilots, always told us that they would airlift us out if we were overrun, but we didn't want to count on that, so we had our own plan.

I tried to sleep more but it was too hot and the smell intolerable, so I got up and took another cold shower. This one was refreshing. Next, I got dressed and even though it was late, I went to the mess hall for breakfast.

• • • • •

Sometime after Johnny came through and I "snapped," I had a harder time emotionally. I was keeping everything locked up tight inside me and was pretty shut down. I also did not believe in the war and felt like a pawn. The conflict roiled inside me. I had agreed to be here and do this job, and yet I knew after the first two weeks that this was all wrong. Something about this whole war was WRONG! I loved the soldiers and wanted to help them, in fact, I was very passionate about helping them. I also stopped going to chapel, felt abandoned by God and was angry that God could let such horrors be done to our guys, the people of Vietnam and their land. I felt like my life was meaningless and had no real vision or hope for any future. I truly believed I would not survive the experience in Vietnam and there was no point in thinking about a future. I did not wear my flak jacket or helmet and seemed to be challenging God — *come and get me if you want me.* I felt it strongly. I was surprised when the year was almost over and I was still alive. I began to ask questions of God: *What will I do with my life? What is my purpose?*

In November of 1967, when the first group of nurses who set up the 12th Evac were leaving, we had a special celebration for them. Since we knew ahead of time when they would be leaving, I wrote home to my aunt, and began to ask for and collect the ingredients for spaghetti. The dinner was for thirty people, so it took some planning. I had our sergeants collecting china plates, silverware, napkins, and glasses from the general's mess. We found unopened OR sheets and used them as tablecloths and began to stock pile tomato puree, tomato paste, whole tomatoes in cans and spaghetti noodles. Those were also some of the things I had sent to me from home, a little at a time, until I had enough for a big vat of spaghetti sauce.

The night before our special dinner, the new mess hall being built was hit during a mortar attack and holes were blown in its side. We were sure the VC got wind of our plans and missed the actual night by one. We were glad they did not hit us the night of the dinner party, or some of our nurses would have been hurt in the attack.

The day of the dinner party, I was in the mess hall kitchen standing on a box in order to reach the top of the pots to stir the spaghetti sauce. The night of the party was a joy seeing the smiling faces of those leaving the next day and those who were saying goodbye to them. We had our chief nurse, Major Douglas, and our chaplain, the executive officer, most of our doctors, nurses and corpsman, and of course our sergeant, present. It was fun to put home-made spaghetti on real plates as they came by to receive their share. We heard some words from our chief nurse, the adjutant and medical service officer, with lots of celebratory shout outs and fun. We took a group picture in front of the wall that was full of holes from the mortar attack the night before.

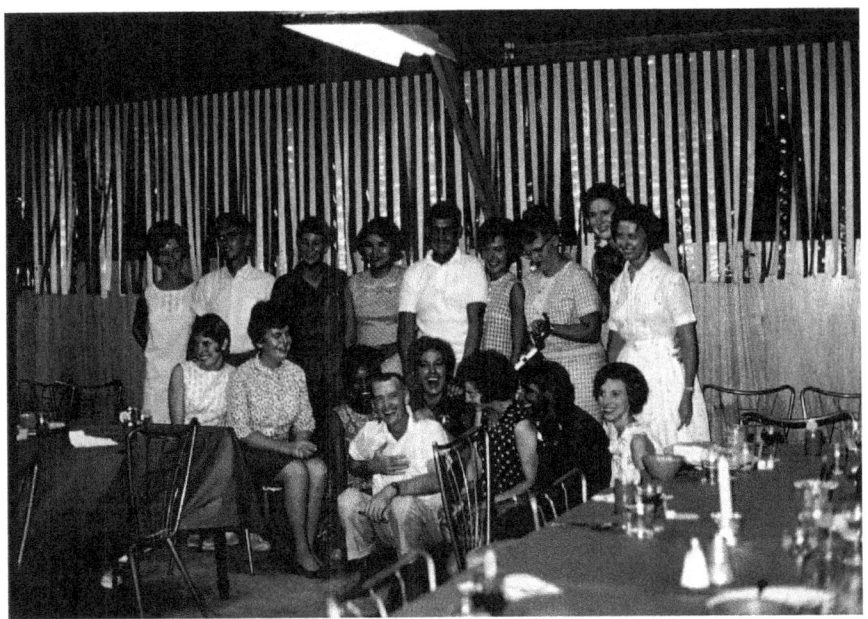

19. Group of nurses, + Dr. Shannon Turney, who built the 12th Evac and are now going home.

The next day we had the 25th Infantry band out playing for the group that was leaving. It was a happy time and a sad time as so many I had been with most of the year were going home and I was staying in the war for another two plus months.

We did write letters home to describe what we were experiencing, but we left out the worst images and any specific locations. I don't know if any of our letters were scrutinized or censored. Letters and packages from home kept us going and all the treats were gobbled up quickly. We all shared what we received with one another.

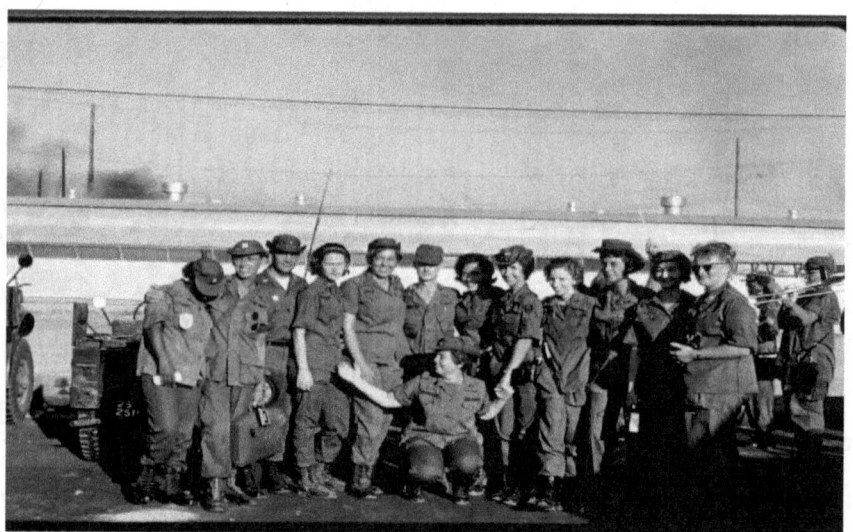

20. Twenty Fifth Infantry Band playing for our nurses and doctors who built the 12th Evacuation Hospital and are now going home.

It was a year of high intensity and pressure to work fast, deal with a continuous flow of casualties and the worst supply system I have ever seen. I heard helicopters, jets, artillery and mortars constantly. I was on my feet in surgery an average of twelve hours a day, some days sixteen to eighteen hours. I was on call four nights a week and was hit with the sights, sounds, smells and horrors of war daily. It was overwhelming immediately, but I could not stay overwhelmed because lives depended on me being fast, knowing what to do, and doing it well. In the beginning, I let myself feel too much and I saw that it would be my undoing if I continued that way. I could not function in those conditions, letting ALL of my feelings be shown and felt, so I had no choice but to shut them down. I learned early on that if my feelings showed on my face the soldiers thought it meant they were going to die.

Many times, I would think these thoughts: *Who will believe all this? Who will know or care? Does anyone know what is going on here? What are the people back home seeing and hearing?* The words and music to, "Where Have All The Flowers Gone?" kept resonating inside me: *When will they ever learn? When will they ever learn?*

It was a year of contrasts, our innocence and the worst horrors imaginable. The beauty of the country of Vietnam, and the ugliness that the war brought, the beautiful people, ours and theirs— first full of life then decimated. The modern day three wheeled vehicles called Lambrettas, the forties style gas station and horse drawn wagons, beautiful peaceful looking blue skies and the sight of gunships and planes bent on destruction and death.

It was a year I would never forget and that forever changed my life. It was a year that hurt me deeply, yet gave me great gifts of strength, resilience, compassion and a lifelong passion for peace and healing.

# Chapter 4
# HOME FROM THE WAR

The day before I was scheduled to go to Long Binh to process out of Vietnam, I heard that Bien Hoa airbase had been hit badly. That was where I had flown into Vietnam and where I would depart from. I was on duty and worked until the day I left. Even though I was going home, the day was emotionally painful for me. I was glad to say goodbye to the most intense year of my life, but I was leaving my friend Claire behind. I was so strongly connected to Claire, Liz, my corpsmen and the entire experience that I could not imagine leaving them all in Vietnam knowing that at any minute they could be killed or maimed for life. There was no question about going home. I wanted to be gone from this place, and yet I did not want to leave behind those I had come to love. I loved them and I loved the 12th Evacuation Hospital. It was probably both the worst and best year of my life. It was the year, more than any other, that changed my life even though I did not fully realize it then.

A helicopter came for me and took me to Long Binh. Tears flowed down my face as I looked at the 12th Evacuation Hospital for the last time and wondered what would happen to those still there. When I entered the bus going to the 90th replacement battalion, I saw that they were the same buses with wire on the windows that started me on this journey. In Long Binh, I was given a private trailer with a shower. It was much nicer than the rat-infested barracks I had when I first arrived in country a year ago. I went through all the army processes to depart/check out of Vietnam and complete my service there.

Waiting for the plane at Bien Hoa airbase that would take me home was excruciatingly painful. I felt like a sitting duck, very vulnerable, as we were all lined up on the tarmac waiting for our "freedom bird." It was obvious everyone there was pretty nervous. As for me, I was terrified.

The VC had hit this airbase with rockets and mortars, the day before we were going home. The airstrip was wide open with no protection. I was thinking, *I have survived a horrific year and now I am fearful that I will be killed while waiting to fly home. What a waste!* I don't think I was the only one who felt that way. When the plane finally came, we were all sweating from the heat and our collective terror and excitement. The plane was a salmon pink color — a Southwest Airlines aircraft. My terror increased as the loading onto the plane was incredibly slow. We were barely creeping forward, one at a time to get on the plane. I felt abject terror being so exposed and vulnerable. What if the VC were to hit the airbase while we were waiting to go home? I wanted to scream and run onto the plane and get out of there!

Finally, I was on the plane and getting settled. When the plane began its liftoff and became airborne there was a huge loud collective intake of air, as if everyone had been holding their breath and were finally able to release it and breathe easy. There was also a collective verbal "yeah!" when the plane lifted off the tarmac. The ride home was very quiet, considering we were leaving the war zone. We all had a lot of intensity, fear, anxiety, questions and excitement. After all, how would it be to return home after such a year? How would our loved ones receive us? How could we ever tell people what we had been through? Would they even want to know? Would they listen if we could and did tell them? Would we be able to relate to them and the world that had gone on while we were at war? Mostly though, it was fear that somehow, at the last minute, something would happen to us that was irrevocable. Fears of the plane blowing up, being shot down, being called back to war, all went through our minds. Getting past those fears allowed space for the excitement of going home and wondering what it would be like.

Many of the soldiers on the plane were in their own private thoughts and feelings, and some were talking to their seatmates about family, hopes and news of the world, and what life would be like "after the war." I was pretty quiet, being the only nurse on the plane — I didn't have a lot to say. I listened and I looked out the window and I thought about all my experiences. The main thought I kept coming back to was, *"What will I do with my life?"* I did not have any plans except to go to my next duty station. Before that I would have a thirty-day leave to go home. I was not excited about returning home, there was nothing there for me. I was excited about going to Los Angeles where I would see my friends Ellie and Bea.

When the plane arrived at Travis Air Force base northeast of San Francisco, it was the middle of the night. The people in charge, whoever they were, would not let us off the plane. I did not know what the problem was, but we were stuck on that plane with all our various feelings and energies for almost two hours. There was some talk that it had to do with not having enough personnel to check us and our bags in, but later we heard it may have been to allow us to avoid exposure to protestors. To have gone through a year of hell, survived the terror of feeling like a sitting duck, and finally get home to America but not be able to touch the ground was excruciating. I felt like a prisoner on the plane, being kept from setting my feet in my home country.

I was tense, angry and very tired by the time they let us off the plane. Once we deplaned, we had to go through a long line and be checked in as customs representatives went through our luggage. I think the fact that I was female may have helped me get through a little faster, because I noticed that they were not very thorough with my luggage and let me go through quickly. I was sure that our guys had previously brought back firearms, drugs and other illegal stuff. It was a long stressful and somewhat agonizing wait. Finally, I was free — and I felt totally lost wearing my class A green uniform. There was no one and nothing to ground me in the experience of being home in the U.S. and not in the midst of the war in Vietnam.

I was free with no schedule, no duty, nothing planned, and not a clue where to go to start. I don't know if anyone else had that experience, but I did. "So now what!" There was no debriefing after a year in war seeing the worse wounds imaginable, no instruction or guidance in how to cope back in the world and nothing from those who sent us to war. I had culture shock, but did not know it. I felt like a tiny dot in the big world of the airport and like a stranger in my own country. I certainly did not experience anyone caring about me when I arrived home after that horrific year. I looked around at the signs and tried to figure out where to go. I knew I wanted to get to L.A., but how do I get to the other airport? It was the middle of the night, about one in the morning and there were few people around.

The climate in January 1968 was very negative toward Vietnam and Vietnam veterans. We were told to take off our uniforms because it was safer for us that way. Safer? This is my country! I was sent to Vietnam by my government, my people. Who posed a danger to me in the uniform of my country?

I had a multiplicity of complex feelings. I was proud of my service and myself, and proud of my brother and sister veterans. Being in life-threatening situations daily created a special bond in me toward those I called my brother and sister veterans. They became like siblings to me and I felt very protective of them. In addition, I hated the war and what it was doing to all of us and to the people and the country of Vietnam. I felt betrayed by my own country and government. I could not understand the feelings of those who were anti-war activists angry with us. It was infuriating that any American would spit on or throw things at us for serving in the U.S. Military. It seemed more appropriate to me that they would be angry with our government for sending us to Vietnam and for waging war there, but not take it out on us — veterans coming home.

• • • • •

In 1983, when an anti-war activist began to yell, shove me around and actually throw eggs at me because I was wearing the uniform of my country — I was devastated, shaken, and enraged all at the same time. A hippie came up to me when I was at a ceremony to honor veterans and said, "You should be ashamed of yourself killing innocent people!" and spit at my boots. She barely got the words out when I returned fire by saying, "You should be ashamed to spit on the uniform of a nurse who helps heal the wounded." I did see a moment of shock cross her face and then turn back to angry, combative, aggressive activism. I was with a male veteran at the time and I was carrying the flag of the United States of America. The other veteran heard other activists yelling, "Baby Killer, Baby Killer" and told me to focus on the flag and keep walking. Later we cried with each other. It is important for people to go out into the streets, march, protest, speak their truth and their wishes and while doing it, they must separate the war from the warriors and honor the men and women who have served, even in illegal/undesirable wars.

• • • • •

When I arrived inside the terminal at Travis Air Force Base in 1968, I eventually found someone who could direct me to a bus that would take me to the San Francisco International Airport. I felt like I was in a fog, or like I was in a dream and everything was shrouded in mist. I had no idea how I got to the red and silver bus however, I did get there. Once on the bus, I told the driver I was going to the International Airport.

As I sat there looking out the window, I saw raindrops on the windowpane. They seemed familiar and friendly. I looked at those raindrops until I became lost in them. It was easy to look at a beautiful clear raindrop as it sat there so quietly and patiently for me to see it, acknowledge it, and join with it. It seemed to wrap itself around me and gave me comfort. I don't know how long the ride was, or anything else about it. I felt so...so... strange. That's it. Strange. But not just as in an odd sort of way, I also felt like a stranger in my own country. The raindrop was familiar, inviting, and it felt like we were old friends. I stayed there lost in the raindrop for the whole ride.

The bus driver said something to me, like the name of the airport or something, to bring me back to awareness of the bus. I did not remember getting off the bus or even going to the plane, but I did get a ticket to L.A. and did get to the plane. I called my friend Ellie from the SFO airport once I knew my arrival information. I asked her to pick me up and she agreed. It would be early morning, 4:30 a.m., when I arrived.

She was already there waiting when I came into the airport and we hugged, went to get the luggage and talked small talk. She told me that Bea was in the hospital and not doing very well, but that she would be glad to see me. Ellie never asked me anything about Vietnam on the way to her home. I wonder if she was afraid to hear the answers, or maybe she was not sure it would be supportive at the moment? When we arrived, I slept.

She took me to see Bea right away the next day. Bea was the practical nurse I worked with for a couple of years before going to Vietnam. She was like a loving mother to me. On the way, I heard a siren and instinctively and automatically dove into the foot-well in front of my seat. I had no explanation. I looked a bit sheepish as I got back up into my seat and Ellie, bless her heart, only looked concerned and never said anything. She kept the conversation going on things about the Sunset Boulevard Kaiser Foundation Hospital where we both worked before I went to Vietnam, and all changes there. After I saw Bea, we went to see some of the people I had known pretty well and looked around the hospital. Ellie and I stopped at a supermarket before I left. I stepped on the pad in front of the door and the door abruptly flew open, which startled and shocked me. My body was not prepared for that jolt. That was my first experience of culture shock. I stayed with Ellie another day before going home to New Jersey.

Once back home, I spent some time with my mother and the aunt and uncle who were there when I was growing up. After that, I went around town to see how it looked, and checked to see if any of my old friends were around. No one I knew and was connected to, was around in Atlantic City when I was there. Before long, I was packing summer clothes and going to Florida to see my dad and brother. It was my brother who picked me up at the Miami airport and drove me to Dad's jewelry shop. I'll never forget how enthusiastic my Dad was about my homecoming, that look in his eyes telling me how proud he was seeing me in my uniform. If that wasn't enough, he would go on and on about how proud he was of me and my military service. His face lit up with delight, and he made sure (as he always used to) that I had something to eat right away. As we sat together and ate lunch he talked about his life, the store and some of his problems. I noticed him smiling a lot when he looked at me and he said, "I am glad you are safely home. I am so proud of you and what you have done. I am giving a party for your homecoming and I invited all the people I know."

"But Dad, I don't know any of those people!" My dad liked to act like a big shot and giving a party was a way for him to do that and show me off. The picture of me in my military uniform was in the window of his store throughout the year I was in Vietnam. He often told people about me, what I was doing, and any news I sent him from the war. I knew the party was important to him, even if it was not to me. The high intensity I was feeling from my year in Vietnam seemed ever present. At that moment in time, maybe especially in the face of the mundane reality being presented to me there in Florida, I was not ready to let that go. It was too important. I had too much invested. Too many memories that seemed ready to bubble over.

Even if it meant that I would, at least for the time, remain dissociated. I didn't want to go to the party but I did since it was at the house. People came up and introduced themselves to me and told me how proud my dad was of me. No one thanked me for serving and no one asked me about it. They drank, ate and talked about one thing or another that was important, or not important to them. Nothing mattered to me. I did not care about any of them or what they had to say; they said nothing of interest. My brother was getting drunk and I went over to talk to him. "Why are you getting drunk? If anyone should be drunk here it would be me, and I am stone cold sober!" He told me about his struggles with dad and the store.

"I feel like there is no future here for me and I am sorry I gave up my career with the FAA. Dad never listens to my ideas about the store, and he is so old-fashioned. It has been hard for me to watch Dad be so self-important and now you are here, and you are the important one to him."

"I get what you are feeling, I know how Dad can be. What are you going to do? Are you going to leave and go back to your career?" As he was unable to answer my questions, I became aware that I didn't feel a need to drink because I was numb and in a fog that nothing seemed to get through. I don't think I was fully there — part of me was still in Vietnam. I was thinking, *I don't know where I belong now. I certainly don't fit in here in Florida and I do not fit in back home in Atlantic City. Maybe I will fit when I get to my next duty station.*

Those experiences were my first in dealing with the mundane world. The biggest and most important thing I learned from that day and something that carried forth, was the conflict I faced in trying to deal with the ordinary. Nothing ordinary or mundane had any value or importance to me after my year of constant intensity, facing my brother soldiers' horrific wounds and potential impending death, plus the threat of death and maiming to me, and those I was close to. I felt the daily challenge of dealing with something that seemed trivial and inconsequential, compared to the intense awareness of mortality and bodily integrity that I dealt with minute by minute in Vietnam. Most of the time in Florida, I laid in the sun, went swimming or bike riding. But despite that sunshine and warmth, despite the blue skies, I remained in that fog the whole time. My thoughts often went to Claire in Vietnam, the hospital and wondering how everyone was doing and what was happening there.

I stayed in Florida until I needed to go back to New Jersey and pack for my next duty station, Madigan Army Hospital (MGH) in Tacoma, Washington. I had requested that assignment while I was still in Vietnam. Linda Howard, one of our nurses at the 12th Evac was from

Washington State, talked a lot about the Puget Sound area in glowing terms describing it as "God's Country." Linda portrayed the beauty of the mountains, the majestic tall Olympic Mountains and the rugged round Cascade Mountain Range. She told me about sailing on Puget Sound and how the salmon swim upstream in the rivers to lay their eggs. She painted a very vivid and inviting picture for me in the short one hour that she and I had during 1967. After asking her some questions, she told me about Pacific Lutheran University (PLU) which was near MGH. She inspired me and gave me hope that I could survive and have a future in "God's Country." I was sold. Every time she said, "God's Country," I knew it was where I wanted to be. Because we could have any assignment we wanted after Vietnam, I was assured that I would go there.

Finally, I was on my way and I was happy. Tom, an orthopedic surgeon with the 1st Air Cavalry, who was stationed at the 12th Evac with me for part of his tour, was kind enough to pick me up at the airport. Tom was married and had been very close with one of the other OR nurses while he was with us. Since he was at Madigan, and I did not know anyone else there, I asked him to pick me up. He was glad to do it and took me to his home at Fort Lewis, helped me find a place to live and got me set up there. He was a good friend and a big help to me in that transition. He also helped me get the position as head nurse of the orthopedic ward. I desperately wanted to get out of the OR, and the army does not like to do that. If you have a specific military occupational specialty (MOS), they want you in it. My MOS was for OR because they trained me to be an OR nurse. I did that to help in Vietnam, but what I liked more was working with the men directly and being able to see and talk with them. In the OR they are asleep and I don't get to interact with them. I told Tom, "Not OR, I want to work with guys who are awake!"

He said, "I am the ward officer for the orthopedics ward. I would love to have you be the head nurse. I will talk to the Chief Nurse of the hospital and request you."

"That is the perfect place for me, thank you so much!" It worked and I did become the head nurse of ward six, the orthopedic ward where Tom was the ward officer. I was in charge, so I was able to create the ambience, structure and rules for the ward that I thought would work best. I loved it. The first rule was that I was the one to greet the bus when the VN returnees came in. It did not matter if I was at lunch or in a meeting, they were to call me when the bus came and I went out to welcome home our wounded warriors. Greeting my brothers back home and telling them that I was a Nam vet and they could talk to me about anything, was a joy for me. It was gratifying to tell them that we would special order any food they wanted to eat, and that we would bring a phone to them if they couldn't walk, so they could call their loved ones.

For the guys who were in traction and would be stuck in bed for many weeks or months, I arranged for them to use our two private rooms. I created a private space for them and their wives or girlfriends. For one entire weekend after their return, they would have the privacy of the room and all my staff had to knock and wait for an OK, to go in. All meals were brought in to them and they had their own TV, and telephone. It worked wonders for them and their morale, since they had already been in bed and traction or a body cast for a long time and had much more time left to go. That arrangement at least gave them some intimacy with their beloved.

After the returning wounded soldiers had finally settled in at the ward, I would check out their wounds and report what I found to Tom. The advantage of working with Dr. Tom, was that we each knew what the other knew from being in Nam together. When I called him, I related the names of the guys, how many there were, what their injuries were and the status of the wounds. Then Tom would order what was necessary for them and come by later to see them himself, add or change anything, and sign the orders that I had already followed through on. We worked as a team and we were unbeatable. I grew to love working with Tom and he with me. Once a week, the doctors had rounds, where they went to each bedside, looked at the x-rays and discussed the case. Mostly it was Tom presenting, since he was the ward officer. It was my job to make sure all the x-rays for each patient were there and were, in fact, the correct x-rays. I also had to have everything and everyone on the ward looking clean, neat and prepared for inspection. The better everyone and everything looked, the better it was for Tom and me, in terms of the army.

When my wounded warriors had conflicting feelings and trouble with relationships, they wanted to talk to me and so I would come to their bed or see them where I could. It was awkward at times because there was no private place. I talked to Tom about that and he arranged for me to use his office on the ward. He had his own office there and at the clinic, which was about 100 yards down the ramp. He said he could use the clinic office and I could use the office on the ward. I did that, and it didn't take long before more and more guys were coming in for counseling.

Many of the guys were having trouble feeling whole because of their injuries and wounds. Some were struggling with understanding the war and its effects on them. There were others that, for no obvious physical reason, had become impotent. All these problems could be connected to their wartime experiences. In Vietnam, they had little to no time off, and their only real outlet for their sexual energy was the young Vietnamese girls who prostituted themselves to provide for their families.

I felt inadequate to help them so I tried to get help and information from the psychologists, psychiatrists, and social workers at the hospital — but I was on my own. No one had time or willingness to help me help the guys, unless they were actively suicidal or homicidal.

In 1968, there was not much I could read to help me either; it seemed that no one really cared enough to provide anything that could be helpful. PTSD was not a known word then, nor was the condition known. It seemed ludicrous to me that in each war, this same condition had reared its ugly head but because they gave it a different name, they tended to forget what they learned and everyone claimed ignorance. In WWI that condition was called "Shell Shock." In WWII the same symptoms were called "Battle Fatigue." The army was not interested in knowing what the condition was or helping vets deal with it. They only cared about the physical wounds.

I noticed that the physical wounds were not healing as expected and I intuitively knew that the reason was the emotional turmoil of these young men. Some had survivor guilt, when the guys in their unit were slaughtered in a crossfire and one guy survived. Others were distressed from having shot and killed people, women, children, or young soldiers. They were overwhelmed by their experiences of being exposed to the threat of death and destruction on a daily basis with no skills to cope with all of it. Many soldiers went on to have a conflict of values that occurred when these sensitive young men were thrown into the horrible situations of war. They would be told to go into a village and clear out the VC. How could they know who was and who was not VC? Sometimes the black pajamas they wore could identify VC, but they did not always wear them. Many times, the VC would lie or a woman would lie to protect them. The wounded American GIs were confused, scared, and could not justify killing because someone was possibly VC. They lived daily with the pressure of walking through the jungle heavily mined or with booby traps all over.

In most of these situations the men felt powerless, and they were. —That powerlessness then took its toll on them when they returned home. They had been in a war far away from their home and the people they knew. They were out of touch with all that went on while they were gone and they came home wounded in many ways that did not show. They were immersed in a very different life as a soldier in Vietnam and were experiencing culture shock and emotional shock, in a world they no longer recognized once they were back home. When their powerlessness manifested in being sexually impotent, it was embarrassing and emotionally painful. They would come to me to talk, yet even had a hard time telling me. After a while, I would just know and say it for them, so they only needed to affirm the truth.

I began my counseling career then, even though I did not know it. We talked about all kinds of things, including their life before the war, their loved ones, their feelings about the war, their activities in the war, and the experiences that were most painful. Eventually, after many days helping them feel more empowered, giving them ways to help themselves and to become self-assured, I would give them a weekend pass. Many times, it was to go out and have a good time and not think about being sexual. Other times, it was to talk with their girlfriend about their feelings and experiences in the war and see how that was received. Eventually, they were all able to overcome it and I always knew the minute I saw them on Monday. I could see it in their faces full of smiles from ear to ear. It was a joy to me to help them in that way and I wondered about the many who did not have someone like me to help them.

I loved those months as the head nurse of ward six and I was good at what I did. Tom and I made a great team and I even grew to love Tom in ways I had not planned. It was one of the patients that actually brought it to my consciousness. He said he could tell by the way I looked at Tom that I loved him, and I did. I even wrote a love poem to him. I knew that he was married and I did not want to break up his marriage. I knew from the time he was in Vietnam until my return, that he was having problems in his marriage. I did not want to add to those.

One night at the officers' club, I shared all this with Tom. He told me he had grown to love me also and he knew me well enough to know that I would hate myself if I acted on my feelings. He cared too much to participate in that. I am so grateful to him for saying that, and saving us both the pain and embarrassment of something we would both regret for all of our lives. We continued to be friends and I dealt with my feelings, while he struggled with his marriage.

There are two young men from that time on ward six that are important. One had his big toe shot off in Korea. He had no place to go and had a long period of convalescence, so I put him to work on the ward. He was very smart, eager and liked doing tasks that I gave him. Because I loved working directly with the patients and did not like all the administrative office work, I began to teach him things like answering the phone, answering basic questions, doing paperwork, and filling out forms and similar tasks. Soon he was a great asset to me and freed me up to be with the patients. He would call me when he needed me and I could trust him to do that. He also protected me from intrusions and harassment from the brass (the officers of higher rank looking for something to focus on) and also warned me when a supervisor was coming. He was wonderful to have there and became invaluable to me and to my patients. It was Toe, as we called him, who was at each bedside the minute someone needed something, and if it was serious, he called me. It was Toe who handled the day-to-day mundane tasks that took valuable nursing time. It was Toe who made sure everything was ordered and in order for all our inspections. He was in that role for several months before he had to report for light duty. It was a mutually satisfying arrangement for both of us and my patients.

The other soldier who was important to me was a young man from New Jersey who had a broken left arm. He was very restless and was not handling being in the hospital very well. I sat with him one day to find out what I could do for him and how I might help him make the most of his hospital time and keep him out of trouble. The latter was quite a challenge, as he seemed to always be in some kind of trouble. He would break the rules and go out drinking or would not take his medications. He would break his cast or he would get the other patients either pissed off or feeling pressured. I learned that he loved to paint and that he believed he would never paint again. I took that information and thought about what I could do to help him. I decided to give him a picture of Mount Rainier to paint. It was a postcard picture of mine that I loved. I bought him some paints, a canvas, and I picked up an easel from Occupational Therapy, then told him to paint that picture for me. It worked and he seemed calmer and had hope. By the time he was finished with the picture, he knew he could paint, he had settled down and was ready to go home on leave, and I had a lovely picture of Mount Rainier.

During the time I was the head nurse on ward six, orders came that awarded me the Army Commendation Medal for my service in

Vietnam. My attitude at that time was very bad. On the one hand, there were many people awarded the bronze star for service in Vietnam that I did not believe deserved it, and there were many who deserved the bronze star and did not receive it. Much depended on the head nurse of the ward or chief nurse of the hospital in Vietnam and who were their favorites, or whether or not they were willing to do the paperwork required in giving such a medal. I knew the value of my service and all that I went through and believed I deserved the Bronze Star, so I dismissed the Army Commendation Medal as not having any value to me. It felt like it was being given to me as a consolation prize and very late. This was March or April of 1968 and I had returned in January of 68. During the ceremony I looked like I felt. My attitude was not very much appreciated. My supervisor came to me afterwards and was angry with me and how that had looked. She let me know by saying, "Captain Blum, you need to change your attitude or there will be hell to pay."

Under my breath I said, "I have already paid hell."

After that, I did soften my attitude, not because of what she said but because of what the patients told me. They understood what it meant to me, and said, "To us, you deserve the Bronze Star, we know what you did in Vietnam and about the politics." I truly loved being head nurse there and doing the work with VN vets. I was sad to leave when my orders came to go to school. Before I left, I was awarded a certificate of achievement from Madigan, which was their highest award. Somehow, I was more proud of that, than the Army Commendation Medal, because I felt I deserved it and was given what I had earned. It is not something that shows, or that I ever said anything about, except on my résumé, but it had meaning to me. Now, when I wear my medals on my fatigue shirt for veteran events, I am proud to wear all the medals that I have. Like many vets, I had thrown the medals out after returning home and then later had to buy them so I could put them on my fatigue shirt or jacket.

# Chapter 5
# THE EFFECTS OF MY VIETNAM EXPERIENCES

In September 1968, I was still on active duty but was assigned to attend Seattle University (SU) for two years, in order to secure my bachelor's degree in nursing. At SU they called me a "retread." That meant I had many years of experience as a nurse and was coming back to school to get a degree. There were six of us retreads, another army nurse and four nuns. We had a blast together studying and playing pool. Often, I was in the basement of one of the buildings playing pool with another nurse and a nun. SU was a Jesuit School; all the teachers were Jesuit priests. I was hoping to work through my loss of faith from Vietnam and spent hours on my knees in prayer in the chapel. I also attended Catholic Mass and other ecumenical programs.

Seattle University was in the central area of Seattle. During the years 1968-1970, when I was there, the Black Panthers were on the march, and there were anti-war protestors burning draft cards and attacking anyone in uniform. I never told anyone that I was a Vietnam Veteran, because I did not want to be the target of anger, rage and the vitriol of the protestors.

I was studying nursing and was specifically interested in psychiatric nursing. I wanted to understand the impact of my own experiences in Vietnam and those of my patients. For some of my practical experiences I asked to be assigned to the Veterans Administration (VA) Hospital. I worked directly with other Vietnam Veterans who had PTSD— during the time the army was beginning to open their eyes and ears to what it was. Because of my own experiences in Vietnam, and since coming home, it was easy for me to understand what the guys were going through and help them. I was also learning basic psychotherapy at SU and using all the new skills I was developing at the VA.

This was also the beginning of healing my relationship with God and creating new friendships. I joined the Chancellor Club, a singles Catholic social group and went to their dances. I met my husband, Joe, at one of those dances in February of 1970. I had been dancing every dance and decided to sit out the next one and rest my feet. I saw this good-looking guy, who had been dancing with a friend of mine whose boyfriend was at the door collecting tickets. Joe came over to the table to ask my friend to dance again. Just as he was about to ask her, her boyfriend arrived and whisked her onto the dance floor. Joe was stunned and stopped in his tracks. He then looked at me with puppy dog eyes and asked if I wanted to dance. I told him I was sitting this one out to rest my feet and then he begged. I finally agreed to dance with him and we fit together nicely. He told me he had just returned from Vietnam and I told him I too was a Vietnam Veteran, a nurse, only back in the U.S. for two years. He stayed with me on the dance floor for the balance of the night and we danced every dance. I had already decided inside myself that I would not go out with him, thinking two Vietnam Veterans together might not be the best choice, but he managed to ask in such a way that I could not say no. At the end of the dance, he asked me, "Are you going to church in the morning?" I told him, "Yes." Then he asked if he could go with me. How do you say no to that? On my way home I thought to myself — *he probably won't show up, because no guy asks a girl to go to church with him, especially a Vietnam Vet.* I was wrong. He showed up and on time. We did go to church together and afterwards he wanted to play Frisbee. I told him no, because I had to study and I thought that would be the end of it. He asked for my number and off he went.

What happened next was another shocker and certainly changed the course of my life. I received a phone call a few days later from a male voice saying he was Lt. Colonel Hart from Madigan Army Hospital. He said that my orders had been revoked and I was to return immediately to the hospital. I started to argue and then realized something was amiss. I said, "Who did you say this was?"

"Lt. Colonel Hart."

"Would you spell that for me please."

"H E A R T." Then I was sure this was bogus.

"OK, who is this? You are not from the military!"

"It's Joe. Will you go out to dinner with me and to see the new Barbara Streisand movie, *Funny Girl?*" When he added the movie, I was in — even though I did not like the way he got to the invitation.

Joe was pretty shabby looking then, with facial hair and an ugly, tan, wrinkled corduroy jacket. I learned from him that he had been smoking marijuana and living part time with a girl across the street from me. As I got to know him better, I offered to help him get cleaned up and focus on his life and what he wanted to do. We went shopping for some sport jackets that fit him and were casual, also some shirts and ties. I encouraged him to get a haircut and told him I would not go out with him if he continued smoking marijuana. I believed that smoking marijuana was a way to not be authentic and feel your feelings. I knew that would not work for me.

When I met Joe, I was in school on the G.I. Bill and had five heavy classes. In March, after dating him for two months, I told him that I had finals and asked that he not call or come over for the three days I would be studying and taking the exams. He agreed and then he came over the second night. He said he only wanted to talk for a few minutes and then he would leave.

He sat on my couch and said this: "I decided I don't want you to be my girlfriend anymore………*long pause*…….I want you to be my fiancée instead." It completely shocked me and at first, during his long pause, I was angry that he would come when I asked him not to, and then say something hurtful like that. When he added the last part, I was stunned speechless.

When I was able to respond, I told him, "You came here when I told you I was taking finals and not to come over. Then you set me up thinking you want to break up and finally ask me to marry you? Are you out of your mind?"

"I think I am in my right mind, thanks to you and I want an answer. Will you be my fiancée?"

"There is no way I can deal with this right now. I need to stay focused, study and pass my finals. Then I am going on the SU Ski Trip to Whitefish, Montana and Banff, Canada. I will think about it while I am gone and tell you when I get back!"

I enjoyed the ski trip and the beauty of the area around Banff and time to think. I thought about what I had experienced in Vietnam and what other Vietnam veterans were going through. I thought about my life and what I was going to do, along with the question Joe asked me. I knew many male veterans were suffering and messed up. I tried to be part of Vietnam Veterans of America but could not take the repeated stories of the guys with so much anger and rage. I was trying to be sane, finish college and keep my faith.

In August 1970, I married Joe and subsequently had two wonderful children four years apart. In 1976, I completed graduate school and became a nurse psychotherapist. By 1980, I had been married ten years my daughter Lorna was nine and my son Sean-David was five.

My post-traumatic stress disorder (PTSD) symptoms began in April of 1975, when the communists took over Saigon. I was full of very sharp relentless feelings about the war and what we Vietnam veterans had been through but I had to shut those feelings down again until early 1980.

While in graduate school at the University of Washington Department of Psychosocial Nursing in 1975, Saigon fell to the communists. We Americans were in Vietnam to stop that from happening, so we had failed in our mission. On that day in April when

Saigon fell, memories came flooding into my psyche, thoughts and images of people and places in Vietnam played behind my eyes like a real time movie. I was devastated! My wall started to crack; the one I put up on the beach at Vung Tau. I was standing in class, in front of a large conference table full of five by seven blue cards flush with information, when my emotions began coming up very intensely. *All our collective losses were in vain*; I completely identified with my brother and sister veterans, alive and dead.

A huge wave of intense emotional energy was rising from deep inside, despair, rage, passion, anxiety, and grief. I ran out of the class and began to walk around the outside of the Health Sciences building, crying, shaking, angry, despondent, and feeling very alone. I know now that I was dissociated again and re-enacting my original angry tromp around the hospital in Cu Chi. Ultimately, I went back in to see my advisor/teacher and tell her what I was experiencing. She and the department chairwoman told me the same thing, "Get your shit together or get out!" It felt like the army all over again. I decided I needed to strengthen the brick wall around my heart. You might think that nursing instructors teaching other nurses to be psychotherapists in 1975 would know a Vietnam Veteran might have some problems dealing with the fall of Saigon to the North Vietnamese. I thought they would be sensitive to that, but they did not have a clue about my feelings or behavior. Their responses demonstrated that to me. I toughed it out.

In 1980, I began to have nightmares and flashbacks. I was already somewhat numb, without awareness of it. I believe that numbness was how I had been coping with my deepest feelings, my life and my marriage. I had a very good friend at the time who did listen to me, empathize and support me. I don't think I would have made it through without her, yet my feelings and needs even became too much for her at that time. She was going through her own struggles and my needs became so great that she had to withdraw her connection from me. She was also a friend of our family who knew and respected my husband, so it was difficult for her to hear the things that troubled me in my marriage, and she became conflicted.

When I told Joe what I was experiencing, he said, "I put all that away on a shelf a long time ago so it doesn't bother me. Why can't you do that?"

As long as I was shut-down I was able to manage my life, but when the symptoms began to break through, I was having trouble both in my work and at home. I was not able to be the wife or mother that I wanted to be. I was not functioning even close to optimum. I was also becoming more and more aware of the subtle changes that had taken place in Joe, as he no longer seemed to be the same guy that I married. It took a while, but it finally dawned on me that this new Joe that I was experiencing was controlling, judgmental, hostile, harsh, critical, loud, and arrogant. He became an attorney after I helped him go through law school, and he often gave me the third degree if my friends called me. "Who is that? What do they want? Why do they want you? What do you know about that?"

Joe would threaten to leave the kids alone when I was at work, if he did not get what he wanted. He also directly threatened my son when he said to him, "If you say that again I'm going to slap your face" or "I'm going to hit you on the head."

Joe used deception and trickery on my son, as he did with me, only worse. He told my son, "Tobacco is poison and will kill you if you eat it!" I learned that one day when Sean-David, age six, looked terrified, his skin was very white and he told me he had a stomachache.

He said, "I ate a piece of candy from the shelf right by dad's chewing tobacco. Dad told me it was poison, so now I am going to die and I don't want to." There was some red powder on the shelf between the tobacco and the candy. Sean-David was sure he was going to die. I told him tobacco is not poison and he would be fine and helped him calm down and feel better. I was very angry that Joe had lied to him to control his behavior.

My own unhappiness at home led me to avoid being there some of the time. When there was an opportunity for me to be somewhere else, I would take it, whether it was to be at work, or with a friend. I almost always came home in time to put the children to bed. I cherished that time with the kids at bedtime, because it was always so sweet, and I was totally present with them. By 1981, it was not so sweet anymore because my husband was very overtly angry and hostile. He would say things to me, or worse yet, to the children about me. He started calling me names in front of the children and making hostile comments like: "The Grinch is home — she decided to check up on us. We have more fun without her." He called me, "sick, stupid, dumb, crazy." He would put the children in the middle, for instance, when Sean-David came to me on Mother's Day to tell me, "Dad did not get you anything because he is mad at you for not doing anything for him for Valentine's Day." As that began to happen more and more, I felt like my self-esteem and my authority as a parent were being undermined and it seemed there was no value in my being there, yet I wanted to be there for the children. I was very stressed about all of that and had an experience that opened me up even more.

I was on my way to work in Tacoma, as a therapist, when I heard on the radio that the Iranian hostages were coming into the airport. They were playing the song, "Tie a Yellow Ribbon Round the Old Oak Tree," and there was a grand celebration for the hostages. I cried and cried nonstop and wondered what they had done to merit such a homecoming when we, as Vietnam Vets, had done so much and received only anger, hatred, name calling, and rejection. It was during that time that the nightmares were occurring about once a week. One of the nightmares was of being in the hospital in Vietnam and hearing the continuous screams of the wounded soldiers. I was also having flashbacks. One flashback occurred while driving on the freeway to work at the Christian Counseling Service. There was an actual army truck in front of me in the next lane. The flashback was that I saw an OD army truck in Vietnam full of wounded and dead soldiers. I saw their dirty faces clearly and their eyes pleading "help me." I began to shake and pulled over to the side of the road.

Soon after that I told one of my Seattle friends about my nightmares and flashbacks. She sent me a very tiny article from the newspaper, about two inches wide and three inches high, which described the first women's Vietnam Veterans' group in the country, starting at the Seattle Vet Center. The woman's name in the article was Jan Ott. I knew her from graduate school, but did not know that she was a Vietnam Vet. Her phone number was in the article and I called her. First, we talked about graduate school and being in the same program, yet not connecting with each other. I was in the family and child pathway and she was in the mother and child pathway at the University of Washington.

Then we talked about her being a Vietnam veteran and she shared her own experiences. Jan had gone all the way to Canada to find two psychiatrists who were trauma specialists and worked in a group format. She went into their group, got the help she needed and then studied with them so she could bring it back here for us. I was grateful for what she had done and what she shared with me. Then I told her my recent problems with nightmares and flashbacks and asked her if she thought the group would help, and most importantly, if I went to the group could I continue to function in my life. I told her about my work as a therapist, my children and marriage and she gave me this answer:

"I don't know how it will be for you. Why don't you come to the first group and then decide if you want to go through the whole sixteen weeks."

That sounded reasonable to me and I decided to go ahead and do that. When I told Joe, he was not very supportive. He saw it as more time away from him. I said, "I am not much good to you or anyone else the way I am now and I would like to feel better and heal. If this group can help me do that, then I want to attend."

He had been very controlling in our marriage, and by this time it had become overwhelming. More and more, my every phone call was being questioned as though I was a witness in his courtroom, slowly taking me to the point where I could rarely talk with any of my friends. My efforts to put him through school soon after we were married were a success, in that he had become an assistant attorney general for the Washington State Department of Ecology, but at home, he had become someone different than that charming man who once had asked me out to dinner and to see *Funny Girl*. Up to now, the abuse had been verbal, but it soon progressed. Joe would not allow any talking at the dinner table, to the point that I could not even ask the children if they wanted anything. He even started to hit my son if he spoke while he was eating. Joe decided what was okay and not okay for me to do when it came to time or money. This group would not cost money, but did take time. He finally agreed to let me go to the first group.

I was scared driving the forty minutes up to the Vet Center. I could not imagine what the experience was going to be like or who would be there. What I did know was that I felt ripe for restoration and wanted to fill up with all the healing I could. I knew something was not okay in me and in my life.

There were eight of us in that first group. We each had a chance to say who we were, where in Vietnam we served, and what we did there. I did not know any of the others except for Jan Ott, one of the two co-leaders. After we had all shared, we were given the opportunity to deal with a trauma from our year in Vietnam. I volunteered to face my biggest one right away; I was ready to go. I had already been feeling and thinking about Johnny, my worst patient and the one that led to my mind snapping while in Vietnam. I was the only one to volunteer.

I spoke up and asked for help to deal with my memories and feelings in relation to Johnny. I was told to talk to him as though he was there in another chair. Jan had put a chair in the middle of our circle for Johnny. This was a new experience for me. Since I was looking for help, I simply did it without question. Jan said to see him in the chair she put in front of me and I did. In fact, within minutes, I could no longer see anyone else in the room. I totally forgot anyone else was there and did not see them — it was only me and Johnny.

Through my tears I said to him, "I am so sorry I ran out on you when you came to the OR to get sewn up. I don't know what happened to me, but I couldn't stand seeing you with so little of your body left. I feel so ashamed that I ran away like that and left you there alone. I don't know how that felt for you and I am so very sorry. I don't know if you survived — or even if you would want to. I wish there was a way to make it up to you, to help you. Can you ever forgive me?"

When I sat in Johnny's chair and expressed what I perceived he thought and felt, (as I was directed to do) he was crying and said: "I am okay now and I was so drugged up when I was on the stretcher that it did not even register to me that you ran out. I just remember looking into your eyes, which seemed to be saying to me what you are saying now — 'I am so sorry you lost so much of your body.' There is nothing for me to forgive, but if you need me to say that, I do forgive you. I am also thankful that women like you were there for those of us who needed medical care. Please stop being so sad. I am okay, I got out of all that mess and you are still in it."

At the time it seemed to take forever and I cried continuously as I talked to him. Writing it here seems so succinct. The counselor was asking me questions to draw things out of me then. When I was done, the others in the room came back into my view. It was as though they were in the dark and only Johnny and I were in a light when we were talking. I had longed for a time to be with him, apologize, and hear what he had to say. When it was over, I felt tremendous relief and knew that I had only just begun the process of healing and needed much more. I was sure that I would come every week and even began to think that sixteen weeks would not be enough. There was so much feeling inside me. When I finally looked around the room at the other women, they all looked numb, stunned, angry, scared, and sad. They had a chance to talk if they wanted to about what that experience was like for them, seeing/hearing me talk with Johnny. Most of them did not say anything. In fact, for the sixteen weeks, I think I got the most out of it. I spoke up every week to do something to heal. Many of the others did not, said very little, and never seemed to challenge me or what I was saying.

One of the most difficult group sessions for me was when I told them I knew there was a cemetery where they buried all the amputated body parts. I even showed them a picture I had of it painted by a solider and in my 25th Infantry Division art book. For years I had a picture in my mind of the burial site for the legs and arms that we had to amputate. I can call up the image of the little wooden crosses in graying wood, and the little gray wooden fence that marks the area... But there is no such place. My mind could not handle the reality, and so made up something easier to accept. One of the women decided to prove to me that I was in denial. She yelled at me, "They threw them into barrels and burned them! Stop lying to us and to yourself." Once again, I felt stunned and shocked. I never knew. Until that moment, I carried the belief and the image of that body parts cemetery. In the group, I was beginning to come to terms with the gruesome reality that all those parts were thrown away and burned.

I was the one in the group that cried the most, yelled the most, and did the most consistent work. Later that would all come back to haunt me. Near the end of the sixteen weeks, I felt like I was just getting started with my healing and did not want the group to end. I feared what I would do when the group ended, because I was feeling more of the emotions I had cut myself off from since Vietnam. Toward the end of the sixteen weeks, we learned about the dedication of the Vietnam Veterans Memorial. That was the summer of 1982. To end the group, we were having a gathering at someone's house and bringing memorabilia and pictures from the war. I brought a set of slides of my experiences, some of which were graphic pictures of surgery.

That night all the other nurses from the group were talking about their trip to Washington D.C. in November. I asked about it, what they were doing, where they were staying. They let me know that they all had plane tickets and were staying at someone's home together. I asked if I could join them and they told me, "You are too sick to go and there may be snipers there, which you couldn't handle." I was pretty devastated by their rejection and closing me out, yet stunned that they believed there would be snipers in D.C. and they were going nonetheless. I felt betrayed by those I called sisters. I thought we were all going through our pain and healing together.

"How could they do this to me?" Because I felt a familial brother/sister relationship with other vets, I thought others did as well. That did not seem true with these women. A few days later, one of them invited me to lunch with them. I thought maybe they had changed their minds and I was both mildly hopeful and cautiously concerned.

At lunch they told me all together, "You are very sick and need help, the slides proved it. How could you show slides of casualties? We are going to the dedication; don't you even think about going because you are not together enough for that." As soon as I heard all that, I left the lunch feeling betrayed again. It felt as if someone kicked me in the gut and I cried and shook all the way home. I did not know what to do, so I called the counselors from the group. They listened but could not do anything to help me.

I had read about a woman in our nation's capital who was a Vietnam veteran nurse and was director of the women's division of the Vietnam Veterans of America. Her name was Lynda Van DeVanter; she was the author of the book, *Home Before Morning*, her own story. Lynda was also featured in an article about nurses from Vietnam talking about their experiences and getting help. I called her, even though it was long distance and very expensive. She was wonderful. She listened and heard about the group, the emotional work I did there, the group leaving me out and telling me how sick I was. She told me that I had probably, "knocked down their house of cards that protected their feelings and they did not like that." She was very affirming, supported me, and the therapy work I had been doing. Lynda told me I could come to DC and she would help me find a place to stay and would meet me there. She encouraged me to come and said it would be very healing for me.

That is when I first started to think about going to Washington D.C. for the dedication. I thought that if I did not go, I would miss out on some important healing experiences. Joe and I did not have the money for such a trip and I did not know if Joe would even support me going. I decided to call my dad, who was a great advocate since my return from Vietnam.

"Dad, I don't know if you heard on the news about the dedication of the Vietnam Veterans Memorial in Washington, D.C. It is happening over Veterans Day this year and I really want to go and I feel like I need to be there. I have been getting some help with my nightmares, memories of the war and flashbacks, and I think meeting other nurses and hearing from the soldiers will help me. Joe and I do not have the money for me to do this, can you help?"

He listened and said, "I will send you the money for a plane ticket." And he did. Then I was in contact with a man named Felix, from Washington State who worked for the State Department in D.C. Lynda had connected us. He offered me a place to stay that was within walking distance of the dedication. He also agreed to meet me in the hotel lobby of the host hotel. Only after all that, did I tell Joe about the trip, that I would only be gone three days and I really needed to go. He was more positive than I expected and supported me going. Maybe he thought I would be done with all of this and we could get on with our lives. I just knew in my heart that I needed to be there, even though I was afraid to go alone. I had never been to Washington D.C. before and did not even know if I would know anyone there. It felt like being at the dedication was deeply important to me, even though I had never done anything like this before with limited resources and plans, yet I wanted to go. No matter what happened, it was still not going to be as bad as my year in Vietnam, it couldn't be.

Joe took me to the airport and was warm and supportive, for which I was grateful. On the plane I met about fifty Vietnam veterans who were from Alaska, Idaho and Eastern Washington — they were all going to the dedication. Meeting them was an unexpected most wonderful gift. We talked together the whole way to Washington D.C. It was great to be with them, talk to them and hear their many experiences and feelings about going back to Washington D.C. I felt so comfortable and at home with them, it bolstered my spirits and emotions. Many had been in vet groups like me. Dave, from Richland, Washington walked with a cane from his war injury and when we got off the plane, he and the other men were getting taxis to take them into town to their hotel. They included me and took my bags. They took care of me and several of them offered me a place to stay. Instead of no place to stay, I now had about four different options and all were free!

# Chapter 6
# THE HEALING BEGINS

It was a three-day whirlwind of activities and emotions. The hotel was full of Vietnam veterans, noise and activity. In the lobby, I met men from all over the U.S. When they found out I had been a nurse in Vietnam, they hugged me and thanked me for what I did. The floodgates opened up and I was crying nonstop. I sat down with a group of them and began asking them how they saw us as nurses and what their experiences had been like. They described the sense of comfort and friendliness they got from just knowing we were there. They told me about their wounds, which hospital they were in and the nurses they remembered. Mostly, they remembered being well cared for and cared about. They also talked about how unsafe it was for many of the nurses, due to the location of their hospitals. Every one of the guys told me something similar to, "You were in the worst area!" That at least validated what I had heard, felt and knew. They had so much love and respect for us as nurses; I had never known or felt that before. I had only been there for a few hours and already I could sense and feel my own heart and soul mending. I continued crying as I was getting hugs from one veteran after another. Their stories were heart wrenching. One man's story, Jed, went home missing one leg and one eye, plus suffered wounds all over. He found his girlfriend with his best buddy who had not gone to Vietnam. He also spent years in and out of the VA hospital for depression. Jed had no happy homecoming from his city or state and felt that his country had betrayed him. He was there at the dedication to meet other vets and get support. Jed felt comfortable telling me his story and he could see how moved I was by him sharing his experiences with me. He said, "That is how all of you nurses were then and now. How do you do that?" I told him it comes from my heart. "You are my brother, of course I care; I love you deeply, feel your pain, and want to help in any way that I can!"

There was a guy who told a common story of his nurse taking good care of him and running the ward very efficiently. He told me about the nurse writing letters for him and his buddies because they could not use their arms or hands to write. Another man told the story of the nurse and her corpsman who had to put all the patients under the beds with mattresses over them to protect them when the hospital was being mortared. One veteran, who had been a Military Policeman (MP), told a story I have never forgotten. This story actually occurred at my hospital, the 12th Evac on the prisoner of war (POW) ward. One of the POW patients, a Viet Cong, was having his dressings changed by the nurse. The VC prisoner reached up and grabbed the bandage scissors from her shirt pocket and was about to stab her with them when the MP shot and killed him. The MP felt proud of what he did and was glad to have saved the nurse. I found out that the nurse is still having trouble dealing with her feelings about the shooting on her behalf.

That same night in the hotel lobby, while sitting with some guys, I noticed an older man wearing a fatigue shirt talking about the Vet Center program. His nametag read 'Blank.' I was teasing him about wearing a false tag leaving the name blank. He seemed to be trying to blend in. Then I discovered his name was Arthur Blank. He was a psychiatrist with the Vet Center program, so the name Blank on his nametag was legitimate. He told us about a PTSD hearing the next day and explained where and when it would be and invited us to attend. My experience of him was very different than with the veterans. There was an immediate bond with each soldier I met. They opened up easily to talk with me and me to them. Not so with Dr. Arthur Blank. He was probably an okay guy, but I did not feel his heart, nor did I feel the connection I did with my brother veterans.

We all went downstairs where they had an expo, a large area filled with booths, information, services and things to buy. Everything was about military units, organizations and paraphernalia. It was then that I finally met Lynda Van Devanter. She was the director of the women's division of the Vietnam Veterans of America (VVA) and was in their booth. We hugged and I thanked her for her help in supporting me and getting me there. She invited me to a party given by *The Stars and Stripes*, told me where and when it would be and that she would be there. *The Stars and Stripes* is the military newspaper we had in Vietnam and that still continues being published. I found an eggshell-colored shirt that had a red nurse caduceus on it and the letters VN on top of the caduceus. I bought it and wore it proudly.

I saw many women wearing fatigue shirts in all the areas of the hotel. I went up to them and asked very hopefully: "Where were you stationed? When were you there?" They would look at me with a blank stare. It was unnerving to me. Each one I approached turned out to be a girlfriend or wife of a male vet. I asked them why they were wearing the fatigue shirt. They were supporting their husband or boyfriend. Maybe so, but it was very painful and frustrating to me. I wanted to meet other nurses who had been to Vietnam. I had not met one yet, other than Lynda.

That night, a group of guys took me to the Vietnam Veterans Memorial (Wall) for the first time. It was dark when we got there and I felt a pull of energy drawing me in as soon as we began walking on the grass in the direction of the memorial.

As it came into full view — it took my breath away. I stood there looking for a long time and then gradually began to walk toward it. The land dipped down gradually as I approached the wall. As I got closer, I saw a woman standing very close to the wall wearing a long winter coat and an OD boonie hat. It is like a sailor cap with the rim turned down all the way around. I stood watching her for a while. She was crying and I thought to myself, *She has to be a nurse. No, maybe she is someone's wife whose husband is on the wall.* She stayed for a while and then gradually she walked in front of other names. *She has to be a nurse, only a nurse would do that.* I felt myself struggling with what to do. I was holding my breath. Finally, I decided to ask/say something. *I can't be the only nurse here.* I also decided, *if she is not a nurse, I'm not going to ask another woman if she was in Vietnam.* I went up to her very respectfully and gingerly and when the moment seemed right, I said, "My name is Sarah. I was an OR nurse at the 12th Evacuation hospital. You look like you could have been there too, were you?"

"I'm Diane Evans. I served at the 71st Evacuation hospital in Pleiku." She smiled and we hugged and cried together. I told her, "I am so relieved to finally find another nurse. I have met many women wearing fatigue shirts but they were all wives and girlfriends of male veterans."

"I'm sure you will see more nurses tomorrow," she said. We stayed together at the Wall for a while and I introduced her to the guys I had been hanging around with. We each allowed our tears to flow more as we looked at the Wall and felt it with our hands. The Wall is an immense upside-down V of black marble that extends out from the left to the right side. The names and dates start going from the center of the upside-down V toward the east (right) from 1959 with the first death in the war, and continue to the end of the east side and then continue all the way back on the west (left) end back to the middle of the upside-down V with 1975 and the last death.

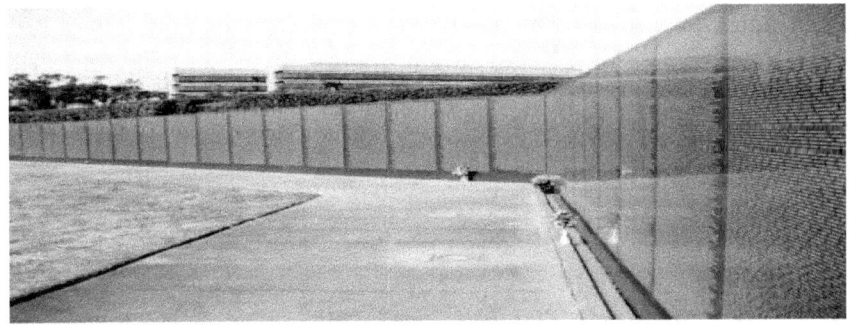

21. The Vietnam Memorial in Washington, D.C.

Because I did not have a single name to remember, I walked in front of the slabs with the dates from Jan 1967 to Jan 1968, 13E-31E. So many deaths in those eighteen slabs of black marble. I went up to the wall and put my hand on it to feel it fully. It felt hot even though it was a very cold November night. Why would it be hot? Is it because it was full of energy? As I stood there crying, remembering and looking at all the names etched in the wall, I knew I did the right thing in coming. We stayed until each of us felt ready to go back to the hotel and we walked back in silence, each of us deep in thought. When we got back, we met a veteran with the book of names and spent an hour or more looking up names, trying to remember names and sharing our feelings with one another.

The next day, we went to Arlington Memorial Cemetery for the Veterans Day ceremonies, and to the tomb of the Unknown Soldier. It was a sunny day. Once there, we found our way to where the ceremony was taking place. It was full. We stood outside and watched the color guard and military band and we saluted when they fired the twenty-one-gun salute. Each time they fired a volley, my body jumped and jerked at the sound and smell of the rifle fire. I was not the only one who had that reaction. There was a man out there from a D.C. newspaper who interviewed some of us and took our pictures. Many of those made it to the paper the day after we were there. Someone gave me a copy of that paper the next day, which I put in an album.

When we went back to the hotel, I gratefully met some nurses. One was Sharon from Alabama and another was Lily from California. I found out that both had been at the 12th Evac Hospital. There were some informal meetings going on among the nurses and when I started to join one of them, Lily took me aside and told me that I was not welcome there. She said there were nurses in there from the vets group I had been in, Nicki and her buddy, Marianne. They were saying things about me to the others like, "Sarah is sick and doesn't belong here, stay away from her" and Lily thought it best I not go in there, so I didn't. I did my best to avoid having any contact with Nicki and Marianne while I was in D.C. I knew that what they were saying had no merit, Lynda had confirmed that for me several times. The way I understood it was that they could not take responsibility for their failure to do their healing work and if they attacked me to cover up for what they could not deal with inside themselves, they felt vindicated.

That night, we all went to the party given by *The Stars and Stripes*. It was wonderful. The first emotional experience was being outside when a male veteran came up to me and asked me if I had been at the 12th Evac. I was wearing the 25th Infantry hat. I told him yes, he hugged me and said, "I thought so — you saved my life!" His name was Mike Rosenthal. He had been in the First Infantry Division (Big Red One) and had been on an operation in our area with the 25th Infantry Division. Mike was hit pretty badly and taken to the 12$^{th}$ Evacuation Hospital. He had been looking for the nurse who took care of him. I told him that I was in the operating room and probably did not take care of him, but he was sure that he remembered me being there and would not hear anything else. From that moment on, he considered me, *his nurse*. He stayed with me the rest of the night and took care of anything I needed. He corresponded with me for years after that, and continues to.

There was a woman outside who was a writer and saw the moment when Mike found me. She came over and asked me to tell her what happened. Mike was standing with me and I told her his story and mine. Her name was Myra McPherson. She was writing the book, *A Long Time Passing*. (Our story is on page 502 of her book.).

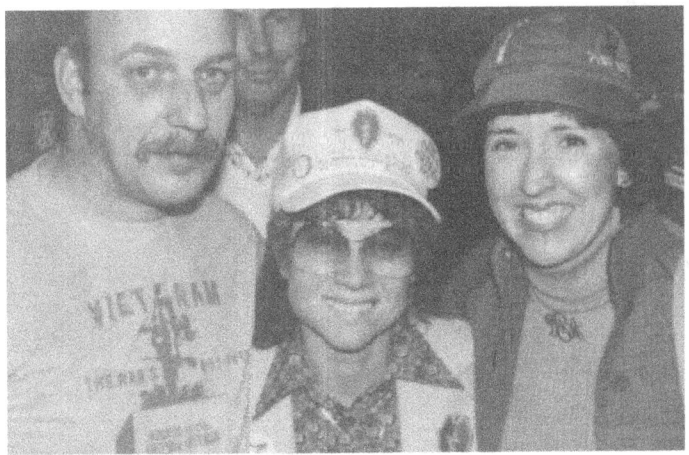

22. Mike on the left and Diane on the right.

We went inside and I found Lynda Van DeVanter with a group of other VN Veteran nurses. We huddled together and started to connect, even though it was very noisy and hard to hear each other. At that point some guys began shouting, "Get the nurses up there," and in the next few minutes some guys were taking us up to the little stage they had in the room. Once up there, the guys began shouting, clapping and saying thank you to all of us. Most of us were crying.

While we were on the stage, we all start singing *God Bless America* and *America the Beautiful*, smiling and crying at the same time. (Not much of a smile from me, reflecting my numbness.) When we finished singing, more and more guys were coming to give me hugs, thank me and tell me their stories. I felt so relieved and happy to finally be with other women veterans and to learn about the effects of my service on the soldiers I went to Vietnam to help.

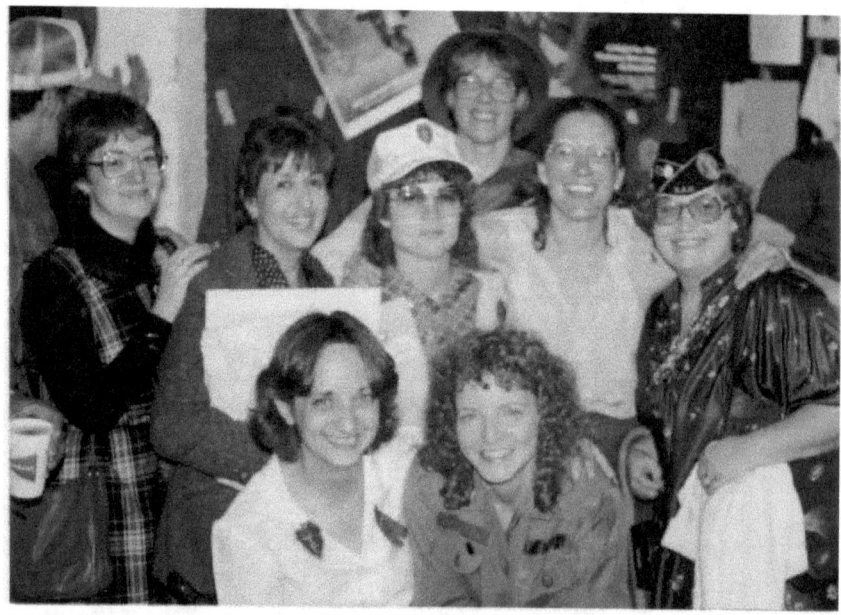

23. The group of Vietnam veteran nurses at the Stars and Stripes party during National Salute to Vietnam veterans November 1982.

I waited fifteen years to hear these men tell me their stories and to thank me. In all those years I did not know how they felt about me or us, or our service. At last, I was hearing and feeling their respect and love and how they perceived us. I heard them tell me I was very courageous and that I/we did a great job. They told us specific ways they were cared for by nurses. Most of the stories were of nurses from the wards because the soldiers were awake then, but in the operating room they were asleep.

I had a great time at the party and felt exhilarated when we left. Mike joined us and we went back to the Wall. We spent some more quality time there and again I cried. This time I did not feel the same need to find women vets, because I had found some already. I simply went from one black marble slab to the next slab, 13E to 31E, crying and remembering. I talked with and supported the guys who were with me as they looked for their buddy's names. When we were done, we all walked back to the hotel and that night I slept very soundly, even though it was not for very long.

The next day, after very little sleep, we all went to the Capitol Building, where the Congress was having a hearing on Agent Orange and PTSD. The best word to describe that experience is *anguished*. I recorded all of it. In the PTSD hearing, I met some other nurses, saw Dr. Blank and heard the words of Dr. Shepherd, who led the proceedings. He presented information that was supposed to give us comfort, i.e., our government was providing the resources we would need to help us resolve our PTSD. I was not comforted nor were any of the hundreds of vets that packed the hearing room. There was standing room only while the rhetoric from the podium was just that, rhetoric — no substance to it whatsoever. They were going around the issue instead of addressing it directly.

The veterans in attendance had experiences of depression, numbing, alienation, insomnia, flashbacks, nightmares, aggression, breaking the law, not holding jobs, and not functioning in their lives. They were shaking and anxious, and felt like their bodies and minds were still in Vietnam. These soldiers were not getting the help they needed. They yelled out to the men with stone faces at the table and the podium. Their pleas, their yells, their cries touched me deeply. I burst into tears many times during the hearing. This was the first time I had heard about the plight of so many veterans in so much emotional pain. The men at the front did not appear to be moved at all. How could that be? The room was literally filled with vets of all types, including women, who were in great pain and anguish. Their pain was palpable. How could those people up there not feel it? My fellow veterans needed to be seen, heard, respected and honored for what they have done and what they needed. Those who were presenting this hearing and who needed to respond seemed stone-faced and numb themselves.

I stood up and shouted out, "Do you hear them? They are in agony. I hear it and feel it! WHAT ARE YOU GOING TO DO ABOUT IT?"

"We are doing the best we can. We have nothing more to say." The room erupted as the veterans collectively shouted, cried and screamed their intense anguish. I was crying and could not believe what was happening. It was 1982, and still the veterans of the Vietnam War and their needs were being ignored. Congress was having the hearing and they said they were doing their research, but they, the leaders, were not listening to us, and they were not providing tangible accessible resources to help us. We were still the forgotten warriors. **Does anyone in this country care that we were sent to war in Vietnam and our inner wounds are still bleeding?** The men in the front of the room seemed like robots.

I was full of feelings and my heart was pounding in my ears about 100 beats a minute. Soon, I was talking with some other women veterans and hearing their stories of pain from lack of facilities for women veterans at the VA. I also heard the stories of men who needed inpatient treatment, which was denied, because the one hospital that provided the needed care was full all the time.

I went from the hearing on PTSD to one on Agent Orange. At the Agent Orange hearing, I was even more ignorant of the issues and problems. I was just beginning to open up to my own pain and experiences and knew next to nothing about any of these issues on a larger scale. The more I heard, the more I was aware of how fortunate I was to be in Seattle, which had resources not available in other parts of the United States.

If the agony level in the PTSD hearing was a ten, on a scale of zero to ten, then in the Agent Orange hearing, it was way beyond ten. The room was packed with standing room only; there were about 300 of us in a room that probably held 250, at most. Senator Tom Daschle and his assistants were in charge and they were listening; I felt their hearts. They seemed to really care. What a difference. They wanted to do more and had been unsuccessful. The Senator and his assistants hoped that through this hearing, our voices could be heard and would fuel their efforts to get us more help and support. Senator Daschle had been to Vietnam and showed us pictures and described the effects of Agent Orange on the people there, especially the children born and unborn. We saw pictures of aborted fetuses that were grossly malformed, and pictures of children who lived with grotesquely deformed bodies due to Agent Orange. He told us that our Department of Veterans Affairs had data, which we could access, which could calculate exactly how much Agent Orange, White, Blue, Purple we were exposed to during our tours of duty. The public only knows of Agent Orange, but there were many more chemicals sprayed to defoliate the trees and thick jungle. Each was given a name based on the color of the band around the fifty-five-gallon drum that held the agent. Nineteen million gallons of herbicides were sprayed over 4.5 million acres in Vietnam. I was personally exposed to 22,271 gallons of Agent Orange, 1,423 gallons of Agent White and 2,339 gallons of Agent Blue. Senator Daschle told us that the Vietnamese scientists and doctors wanted to work with ours to learn more about the effects and what to do about it. We were reminded that our government was still not interested in acknowledging that there were damaging effects on our children and ourselves because they did not want to have to pay for treatment and compensation. Senator Daschle and his staff were still trying to get some legislation through so that veterans could be evaluated and treated through the VA system for exposure to all the toxic agents.

The veterans stood and told their stories one by one. A guy from Florida took off his shirt and showed the senator his side and underarm, where he had a burning rash that had been there for years, and no one in the VA would acknowledge that it was related to Agent Orange. Another vet was crying and telling the senator about his child born without a kidney and with a blood disorder the doctors were saying was from toxic chemicals. Yet another vet was shouting and crying while telling the senator about his sarcoma. He was not getting any help from the VA even though the literature identified sarcoma as related to dioxin exposure. I heard story after story of the agony and anguish of my brother and sister vets and their children aborted or born with grotesque deformities.

"We lived with it, we slept with it, we bathed in it!" screamed one of the vets. "We don't want money, we want accountability and acknowledgement that our government did this to us! **We don't trust you**! We want treatment for our children and our bodies." I heard my brother vets' excruciating anguish and I was sobbing while my tape recorder recorded everything. Once again, I was stunned and then scared as I started to think of my own children.

My husband and I were both Vietnam veterans. My daughter had recently seen an orthodontist who told me the stains on her teeth were from toxic chemicals. He asked me what she was exposed to. I thought of the ear trouble my daughter had when she was younger and the problems with her eye. She had a congenital paralysis of the nerve that went to the muscles of her eye, which limited movement, and the pupil was permanently dilated and the lid drooped. I thought of my son, and the trouble he had with his eyes, ears and bowels.

When the hearing was over, I happened to be in the elevator with Senator Daschle. I asked him if he thought that the problems my children had could be from Agent Orange. He said "most certainly" and suggested I get letters from the doctors and orthodontist to verify what I was saying and send them to his office. He gave me his card. As we were getting off the elevator, I was in a state of shock, numb, my mind a blank. Before that moment, I had not considered the connection between the conditions of my children and Agent Orange exposure. When I could think again, I would have a lot to consider. (I was later denied any help from the VA for the conditions of my children.)

The next day was the big day. They called the event the National Salute to Vietnam Veterans, which included the parade and the dedication of the Vietnam Veterans Memorial. I did not know what to anticipate except that I had to be separate from the nurses I had met there and the guys I was hanging out with because we would be marching by state. Fortunately for me, Dave from Richland, WA, the Vietnam Veteran I met on the plane coming to D.C., and Felix, the man who worked for the State Department, were both from Washington. I finally got to meet Felix in person and was introduced to a guy named Joe, who was working with a vets group in Seattle. We stayed together on the Capitol Mall grounds waiting for the parade to start. This was the very first ever parade for Vietnam veterans, seven years after the end of the war, and for me fourteen years after my return home. I did not know how to respond and was not sure what to expect — yet hoped deeply that it would all be positive. They gave us a pin to wear that looked like a small replica of a service medal and it said National Salute to Vietnam Veterans. I felt proud to wear it.

I had come on this trip with only slacks, blouses and a raincoat. A veteran from the 25th Infantry Division gave me a hat with a patch on it; the yellow lightning bolt on the red background that represented "Tropic Lightning," the call name for the 25th Infantry Division. This symbol is sometimes called the "Electric Strawberry." I wore the hat with my pin on it and I had my caduceus pin on the lapel of my tan raincoat. I was not wearing anything to identify me as a Vietnam Veteran Nurse except those items. That is how I marched in my first ever parade of honor as a vet. The parade was in 1982, and I served in Vietnam in 1967.

I was proud to march with the state of Washington, where I landed after Vietnam and never left. Because I was so short, only five feet, the guys put me in the front row, although there were not many rows because few of us actually came from Washington State. The parade was amazingly wonderful and healing. As we marched down Constitution Avenue there were people lining the streets. Many had signs saying "Thank You" and they waved flags and shouted "Thank You" and "Welcome Home." Some even saluted us with their hands. I cried so many times I lost count. I was truly touched to receive their heartfelt thanks and respect for us, and what we had done. As I received their shouts, waves and smiles, I began to feel less vulnerable and started to smile back and I began to put my right thumb up in the air to acknowledge them as an emotional "YES! Right On!" It was a very uplifting and truly healing experience for me.

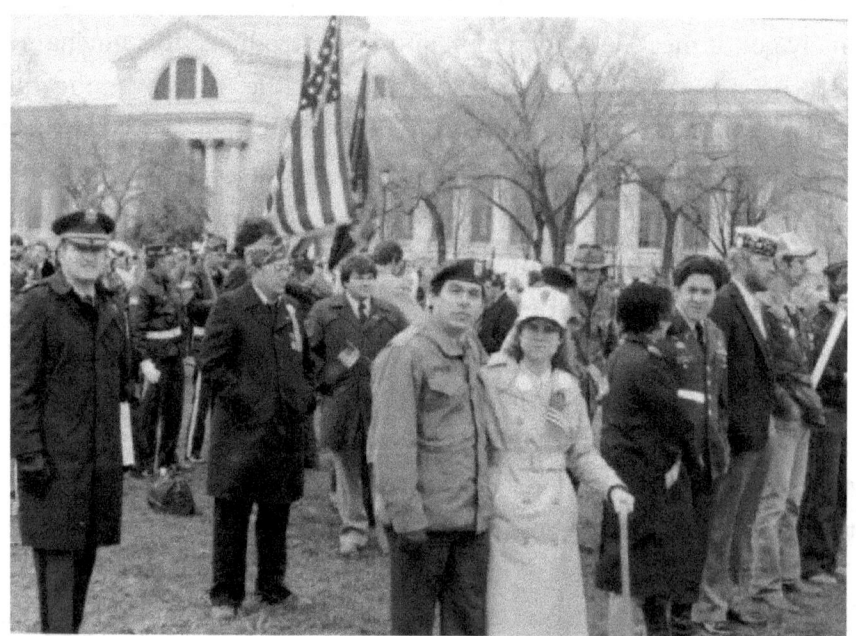

24. Joe in red beret'next to me then an unknown woman and Felix at the start of the parade.

When the parade was over, we milled around for a while and then gradually made our way onto the area called, the Mall. That is the large grassy area that extends from the Capitol Building down to the Lincoln Memorial. We wanted to get as close to the Wall as possible. Once I got there, I found Lynda Van Devanter and some other women vets. We decided to hang out together and while we were there, a guy came up looking for a nurse. He talked about being in a long-range reconnaissance patrol (LRRP). He was wounded and taken to the 12th Evacuation Hospital for surgery and recovery. It turned out that he was wounded during 1967, so he latched onto me, gave me a big hug, cried and thanked me. I must admit there were moments like that when I did not know what to do or say. I did not know if I was a nurse who cared for him. I could not remember any soldiers' names, and did not even know their names when in surgery. He may have come through and been on the OR table when I was there, or he may have had a different nurse. I do not know if it really matters and yet for me, it was difficult to take credit for something that I may not have done. I accepted his hug, his heartfelt feelings, his tears and I listened to his stories nonetheless. I felt very connected to him emotionally at the time and yet inside, I still had doubt. *"Was I really the one, is it right for me to receive this from him? It feels good to hear him share his gratitude and positive feelings toward us nurses."* All of that was going on inside me all at the same time. He stayed with us for the rest of the day and then I never saw him again. I will never forget that poignant experience.

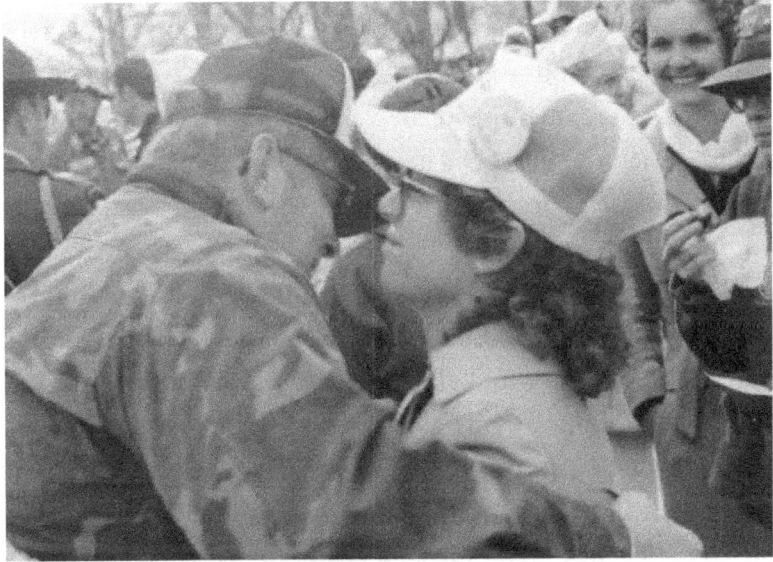

25. LRRP veteran who thought I took care of him when he came to the 12th when wounded.

As far as I could see, there was an ocean of people flooding the Capitol Mall. I would guess thousands of Vietnam Veterans, their families and friends from all over. It was a gray, cloudy, overcast day and there was a balloon of the American flag flying above the crowds. The air was electric with excitement and the energy was very high, an energy of anticipation, sadness, anger, rage, and anxiety from the vets. We waited for several hours for the ceremonies to begin, and in that time, we talked, snacked, laughed, cried, remembered and met other vets. When the ceremonies actually began, we were within about 100 yards of the stage. We could see some of it and hear it very well; loud speakers were set up all over the mall. It seemed incongruous to me that all the vets were outside of the ceremonial area and the dignitaries were inside. I thought they were honoring us, the vets. So, why were we on the outside of the fence? I was not healed enough at the time to be outraged by this, but by 1993, when they dedicated the Vietnam Women's Memorial, I was, and a group of guys lifted me over the fence so I could be inside while I watched the dedication of what I refer to as, "Our Memorial."

When the ceremony began to dedicate the Vietnam Memorial Wall, the speakers were good — they made us think, they were inspiring and yet every time they mentioned the veterans they said, "The men who fought! The men of courage! The men who gave their all!" Except for Brigadier General George B. Price, there was not any real mention of, or recognition of any women who served in Vietnam. He acknowledged us women who served well. That discount continued to prevail for many years and still does to this day. They dedicated the memorial and then we could all go up to it and do our connecting and grieving. With the thousands of vets and people there, it took a long time to get close to the Wall itself. When we finally got up close, it was near dark. The crowds had thinned considerably by then and we had time to look, listen, feel, and to hug each other. We did all of that for each other and for those who we did not know. We saw many letters, poems, pictures, flowers and military medals that were left there by people who visited. We stayed there for hours reluctant to part company, until we knew we had to go back to the hotel to say our goodbyes and sleep.

The next day I flew back home and I cried on and off the entire flight. I felt like the flood gates of grief were opened up. I felt as though my tears would continue to flow forever. I simply could not stop crying. What brought it up was finally meeting guys who could tell me the truth about their experiences with nurses. That and being acknowledged, hugged, connecting with others, and floods of memories from my year in Vietnam began the healing for me.

Unlike the trip to D.C., I was not with a group of vets, I was alone and all I had were my memories and feelings. I remembered and felt my grief the entire seven-hour flight home. When I was home, my crying and sobbing continued. It was as though a zipper had been pulled down my torso from my heart to my lower abdomen and everything inside was pouring out of me. I did not know what I could do except feel them. I did not go back to work right away and Joe was gentle and comforting to me for a while. The children were sensitive in their own ways and knew that something was different about me, in addition to my obvious crying.

I think it took me about two weeks to stop crying continuously and return to periodic bouts of crying. I went back to work and resumed my life, yet my life was never the same after that. From that opening, all of what I had built up around my feelings and my heart began to disintegrate, even if I was not aware of it at the time.

In 1983, when they finally put an American flag at the Wall to honor our brother and sister vets who died in Vietnam, Joe and I went back to D.C. to stand in a three-day vigil at the Wall. Many people do not know that our Vietnam Veterans Memorial did not have a flag on it for over a year. In 1982, after the dedication, many male Vietnam Veterans were angry and felt they were being discounted again. Their own country deliberately omitted the flag from the memorial. The shame many felt was exacerbated by that slight. A group of vets found a flag on a government building and literally took it from there and brought it to the memorial. From that moment on, there were always Vietnam Veterans standing on top of the Wall holding the American flag. During our part of the vigil our group from Washington State was standing with the flag over three days and nights. I also joined the Vietnam Veterans of America, VVA, and ran for a position on their first board of directors. I wanted to do something more to help veterans. I gave an inspiring passionate speech and was elected, along with Lily Jean. We were the first two women elected to that first VVA Board and both of us served at the same hospital, the 12th Evac. Getting anything done while on the board was a challenge because everyone had big feelings and lots of words to express but that did not lend itself to making decisions and acting on them. I was frustrated by that many times.

It was also stressful because there were some terrible things happening that we were discussing, horror stories about the mistreatment or poor treatment of vets in the VA hospitals. There were vets who were laying in wet beds, falling out of bed, having urine bags overflow and having pain medications withheld. Our Vietnam Veterans experienced the worst mistreatment and nursing care ever reported at the VA and the legacy of that led to many, including me, avoiding the VA for thirty to forty years.

It was a very busy two years on the VVA Board, because I was flying back and forth to Washington D.C. once a quarter. I took on the task of trying to get legislation passed to study the effects of Agent Orange on women veterans and their children. I knew both of my children had been affected and I heard at the hearings how many vets were suffering from the effects on them and their children. My daughter's eye and eyelid were not normal from birth and she had several surgeries to correct it. Her ears were affected as well, and to this day she never knows when she will experience extreme vertigo. My son's bowels and ears were affected for the first ten years of his life and he was in pain. Other veterans' children had nonfunctional or missing kidneys, born without limbs, or disfigured. The only studies done at that time were on the men who actually dropped Agent Orange from airplanes.

Women veterans were never important to the military, the government or the VA, (we were never even counted — they literally did not know how many women served in Vietnam) and certainly they were not important enough to study for effects that the government would rather not know about. I went to get support from congresswomen Marcy Kaptur and from scientific groups. I managed to get a bill drafted and supported, but at the last minute they tacked it onto an omnibus bill, and when that bill was defeated, with it went our hopes for a study. It was two years of work unfulfilled in outcome.

Toward the end of my term on the VVA Board in spring 1984, I was beginning to feel ill. My term on the board was to end in November. When I began to feel sick, I decided that perhaps a massage would help. I had the name of woman who did massage in Seattle and went to see her. She took one look at me and my body and said that she could not massage me because my body was too toxic. She told me to drink only lemon water for three days and to go see Dr. Johannes Lui, a Chinese doctor only considered an herbalist in the U.S. I did as she suggested and sought out Dr. Lui. He was a short Chinese man who did Chinese Health Assessments and prescribed diet and herbs. He looked at my tongue, eyes, and hands, felt my pulses and took my history. I had my yearly physical only a week before and the results of my pap smear revealed a small spot of cancer on my cervix. I told that to Dr. Lui, along with how I was feeling. He then asked me if I had been exposed to anything toxic. I could not think of anything (still not connecting to Vietnam and Agent Orange). He said that toxic chemicals had affected me. That is when I suddenly realized it could be Agent Orange. I told him what I knew and he shook his head and went on from there.

He gave me some herbs to brew as a tea to drink every day and he sent me to a Chinese store to buy some little black pellets that were to clear out my liver of all the toxins. He also wrote out a list of what I could and could not eat. I was to eat mainly brown rice and apples after I poured boiling water over them, and I could eat oranges. I was to return to him in three weeks. In the meantime, I was scheduled for laser treatment for the cancer. I went to the day surgery center at Virginia

Mason Hospital in Seattle and was there only a few hours. It was easy enough, quite painless and quick, with only a short recovery from the anesthetic after which I felt fine. That was only the physical part.

I knew that I had created the cancer of the cervix by my constant thought, *I can't live like this*, in relationship to my marriage. I had been repeating that thought with desperation for at least two years. I felt that was the way I created the cancer, even though it was not conscious as I was doing it. The thought, *"I can't live like this"* was what I felt and kept repeating. Now it had manifested in actuality. I was frustrated and sad about my life, not feeling happiness or joy, feeling alone and isolated, even though married. I was even considering killing myself because I was in so much emotional pain and did not know how to change my experiences to feel joy rather than despair.

# Chapter 7
# PTSD AND HEALING

There was a point earlier in the year when I was very depressed and seeing a therapist who told my husband Joe not to leave me alone because of my suicidal thoughts and inclinations. On one of my worst days, Joe left me alone. I called a colleague to come and be with me. I knew that I was not safe to be alone and it was clear that Joe did not take that into account, even though my therapist had told him not to leave me alone.

I went through two therapists and was still not getting what I needed. My first therapist was not hearing me or connecting deeply enough with me. The second one had a political agenda and wanted me to go out and promote her anti-war agenda. I was far from being able to do that. I continued to struggle in every way except with my own work as a therapist.

In May 1984, I had been searching for a therapist to help me and found a former teacher of mine from undergraduate school, Elaine Childs-Gowell. She was one of my favorite teachers from the University of Washington in 1970. I attended a clinical training she was giving, and after the workshop, I asked if she remembered me and if she would see me as a client. She did remember me and agreed to work with me. We met for several months when I was very deep in my anguish, pain, and confusion about Vietnam, my life, my marriage, and was probably in the worst of my PTSD. I was not easy to be around because I was very needy, anxious, unsure, depressed, disconnected, having flashbacks and nightmares and I was very angry. I really needed therapy and was very ready for it. I had also just come out of a three-day spiritual retreat, getting clear about my marriage, my life and what I needed to do to move forward to be healthy and happy. My guide at the retreat helped me see how unhealthy my marriage was. I was asked to list all the healthy and unhealthy aspects of my marriage. As I wrote the lists my body became colder and colder. I was staring at a very short list of healthy aspects and pages of items that were unhealthy. The reality was sinking into my mind, emotions and my body.

During my time at the retreat, I became conscious of many things about myself. The first was how deeply impacted I was by simply having a room of my own and feeling safe within it. I felt contained, warm, held, and I had privacy. It was my space. I was not aware at all that I had been missing that until I went to the retreat and actually had my own room. It was a big "aha" moment for me. I also had silence and that too was missing in my life. Joe was very loud when he walked and talked, and of course having young children did not allow for much quiet. At the retreat, I had time to walk in silence, write in silence, and be in silence, all of which resulted in a new clarity that I had never known before. I was ever so grateful for my time there and the help I received. I had time to *be*, to reflect, to feel, to open up spiritually, to pray, to understand, and to write what I knew and felt. I wrote a poem on that retreat called "We Did It All For You."

In remembrance of so many of us nurses and what we experienced.
Dedicated to so many of you, soldiers of an unwanted war.

WE DID IT ALL FOR YOU ©
We heard about you on the radio,
We saw you on the TV.
We knew you were hurting so,
We went to the Nam Country.

We took you as you came,
We felt the mud and dirt.
We knew we would go insane,
We knew we couldn't stop the hurt.

We tore off your fatigues and boots,
We searched your parts and your holes.
We saw your limbs torn off like roots,
We suffered with you, for all our souls.

We stood for hours in your lost blood.
We screamed inside at those awful sights.
We cursed and raged and slid in the mud.
We knew the results of your frustrated fights.

We held your hand and said to hang in,
We prayed in silence for your sweet life.
We knew full well our country's sin,
We hoped in vain for an end to strife.

We went to be with you and help you too,
We weren't prepared and neither were you.
We couldn't believe what we all went through,
We worked to heal but who ever knew?

We pumped the blood and helped you sleep.
We changed your dressings and cut the pain.
We turned you over and scrubbed your feet.
We talked and listened and went insane.

We couldn't cry - or we couldn't work,
We tried to be calm to do our job.
We never knew where the enemy lurked,
We daren't let out, even one sob.

We sorted you one from another,
We chose - do you live or die.
We struggled so much for you our brother,
We knew in our hearts we needed to cry.

We were beside you in the operating room.
We cleaned your wounds and put you to sleep.
We cut and sawed from noon to noon.
We swallowed and choked and sighed so deep.

We saw you at your very best, proud and smart.
We saw you at your worst, torn and wounded,
We held your maimed and mangled parts,
We lifted, pulled, pushed and turned your head.

We yelled for supplies that we didn't have,
We cringed when we read the media lies.
We held our breath as we applied the salve,
We wondered when America would open her eyes.

We hated the mud and rain and dust.
We hated the protests and lack of support.
We drank and danced and how we cussed.
We hoped and prayed for the war to be "short."

We wondered how you did perceive us,
We worried how well we were really doing.
We came to help, to heal and not to fuss.
We couldn't control the ugly war we were viewing.

We felt angry, enraged, sad and sick inside.
We wanted to protect you from anything more.
We didn't understand and we wanted to hide.

We couldn't leave you, we were all in a war.

We were frustrated and mad at all the news.
We hoped in vain for the telling of the truth.
We found some solace in beer and 'moody blues,'
We took pictures of war to record the truth.

We didn't all make it, and neither did you.
We became numbers, counts and stats!
We were killed and lost, and wondered who knew?
We were people - but were counted like rats!

We came home in the dark, broken or boxed.
We were the shame of this Country we served.
We were attacked or shunned like we were poxed,
We whores and dykes, names so undeserved.

We loved America and you dear sweet brothers,
We were nurses true blue and oh so few.
We cared, we suffered Nam sisters and brothers,
We want you to know – we did it all for you!

©Written by Sarah Leah Blum, May 1984
Operating Room Nurse
12th Evacuation Hospital
Cu Chi, Vietnam, 1967

When I felt better, I began to process my feelings about leaving my marriage and planned how to leave. One day in February, on my way to a therapy appointment with Elaine, I had one of my worst flashbacks. It was snowing and I was driving on the freeway to my appointment. A white truck in the lane in front of me was swerving. I instinctively moved away from it and kept watching the truck. It swerved into the guardrail on the left as I moved to the right. As the truck hit the guardrail I flashed back. The truck in my flashback burst into flames and I heard the sound of mortar fire. I immediately began to panic; my hands squeezed the wheel and I was struggling to breathe. The white truck on the freeway hit the guardrail and slid sideways. Somehow, I was able to get off the freeway at the correct exit, only a few miles from where I was at the time. When I saw Elaine, I was fighting to breathe and talk. My breathing sounded like croaking, with very harsh raspy sounds. She was able to help me calm down and get back to being clear and grounded by the end of the session.

I went through therapy with Elaine for four- years from 1984 to 1987. In that therapy I went as deeply into my past, my body, my feelings and my soul as I could. I dealt with the worst experiences of Vietnam, releasing immeasurable amounts of anger, rage, fear and anxiety from my military experiences, my marriage, and my childhood. I learned to go into each experience fully with my body and my feelings, do what I needed to do, and then come back out of it and be stronger and healthier. I kept putting off doing what I referred to as my, "Vietnam work," because of fear. I felt like I had a time bomb inside me that was going to go off and I did not want anyone to be hurt by it. I could not verbalize that at the time, so I would simply avoid doing what I knew I had to do.

Then one day in group with Elaine, I was ready — and decided to dive in. It was like standing on the end of a diving board, terrified that once I dived in, I wouldn't come back up and out. I knew I was going into the anger, rage, terror, despair, and craziness that had lived inside of me for about twenty years (it was now 1987). I took a good look around the room before I started and then verbalized the question to everyone in the group, "Are you going to stay with me through this and be here when I come back out?" They all nodded yes. I was on my knees with a large pillow in front of me and I allowed myself to go all the way into those intense feelings that had been walled off for so long. I yelled, screamed, cried, punched and pounded the pillow with a tennis racquet and let it out. I released a lot of anger and rage toward our government and the VA and toward the experience of being in the Vietnam War. I cried my salty bitter tears of grief for all the many young men who were slaughtered and the loss of innocence so many of us felt. I expressed the deep enduring pain of the devastation the war wrought on us, the Vietnamese people and the land, and released the terror of so many times when I thought I was going to die. I know this went on for a long time, maybe twenty or thirty minutes and when I was drained, wet with tears, eyes swollen, nose full and voice weak from screaming, I looked up to see my group members. They all looked white — like ghosts, and their bodies were pushing against the wall behind them as though trying to escape. I was spent and sat there looking for a while before I spoke. My first question was, "Is anybody breathing?" And then I heard the strong intake of breath from many of them. They had been holding their breath. Then we talked about what that experience was like for them and for me. That was the key healing experience for me, among the many other restorative processes. I felt safe and supported in whatever I needed to say or express. I discovered I could dive into the worst of what was inside me and come backout feeling and being better than before I went down into it. I could survive the worst of my wartime experiences yet again.

Having acceptance and support was invaluable to me. I could share anything there, even the shame I felt when I ran out on Johnny and when I shot a gun from a helicopter at those I thought were VC. I had so many intense feelings about what happened to those young men, my brothers, and so many questions. Once I began, I did not want to stop until the feelings were all gone from inside me. I worked week after week to release them. Once I had done that there was space for the good stuff of life, for joy, peace, connections, freedom, fulfilling my needs, relationships, a vibrant life for me. I filled up the empty place in my heart with love, peace, God, and I learned how to communicate authentically, clearly and powerfully. I believe what supported me in doing all that was having others be there with me. I was seen, heard, affirmed, and validated. Elaine and the group members were authentically there supporting me, were outraged with me at some of the experiences, and nurtured me when I needed that. I could be completely myself with all that I felt and thought, and be accepted and loved. That constant, supportive, loving container made it possible for me to heal. I used that container to do the therapeutic work I needed and I freed myself of PTSD.

I was so impressed by the therapy and how powerful and effective it was that I later became a student of the process and Elaine became a teacher and mentor. I had many small group classes with her, case reviews, and I began co-leading groups with her. By 1986, I began leading my own groups and working with other veterans who also left their PTSD behind, and live healthy, active lives today with no sign of PTSD. The VA has a different approach to PTSD. They believe that their job is to manage the symptoms; they have no idea how to help a veteran actually heal from PTSD and leave it behind. It could be done! I had done it myself, and now I do it with and for other veterans, and people traumatized as children. PTSD can be healed. That does not mean you will never be triggered but if you are triggered, you know what is happening and have the tools and people to support you returning to your healthy, grounded, clear, competent self.

Back in 1985, while I was focused on my own healing and that of my brother veterans, I connected with a Vietnamese hospital worker called Thu Van Nguyen, who was also working on healing for her community of Vietnamese veterans. Together we began to share our passion for healing and our vision for how to do that.

We came up with a plan to bring all the veterans together in the Veterans Hall at Seattle Center on Veterans Day 1985. We called it Recognition/Friendship Day. There was a lot of opposition from all of the American Veterans organizations. They were not yet healed and were still hurt and angry at what took place in 1975 and how they were treated when they came home. Many would call me or Thu and threatened us if we went ahead with our plan. I understood their reactions and believed they needed what we were proposing but they did not understand the value of it. I spent a lot of time supporting Thu Van Nguyen when she was frightened and wanted to back out. I stayed positive and trusted that it would all work out well if we could sustain ourselves and what we believed.

When the day finally arrived, it was one of the most healing and emotionally moving events that had taken place in support of our Vietnam and Vietnamese veterans. The Veterans Hall was packed and had standing room only. Every Seattle newspaper and TV station was there, and they had a lot to report on. We brought in the flags ceremonially, and then I opened up the proceedings by sharing my story of being a nurse at the 12th Evacuation Hospital, Cu Chi, Vietnam and my vision for healing all of us, both American and Vietnamese veterans. Then Thu shared her story and vision. From there, we alternated the sharing of stories, one American and one Vietnamese.

After the first set of soldiers' stories, the two men hugged each other and cried together, and that continued throughout the event, story after story, followed by hugs and crying. The men began to understand there was plenty of pain and suffering to go around. It was time to heal, and they began it that very day.

# Chapter 8
# UNDERSTANDING PTSD

No one description of PTSD can fit every person. We are all unique, have different personalities and expressions; and we have had different external and internal experiences. It is likely that no one responds to the same trauma in the same way. One person might go through an experience and not be traumatized or even consider it a trauma, yet another can be devastated by the very same type of experience. It is a matter of perspective, past experience, meaning and sensitivities.

As I struggle to write this, I see why it is so difficult. If we only focus on perspective, which in itself encompasses how many different people there are in the world, we get millions of different views. However, if we talk about past experiences, we find that to be the number of people multiplied by the number of different experiences each one of those people had. With that unwieldy number, we shift to meaning and multiply that by how many potential meanings could be garnered from each one of those different past experiences. It feels like we are caught in a quagmire. Among the different people with different perspectives and meanings, we have some with specific sensitivities. I truly believe some people have what I refer to as sensitive souls. I have never come up with any better words to describe it. It is true for me and for others I have known. It is not to say that those of us with a sensitive soul are not also resilient and strong, it is a certain way that we experience and tune in. It might be connected with compassion and being compassionate. For those who care deeply about other people and other life forms, we/they tend to be sensitives. Anyone in that category is likely to experience the deepest hurt and pain to any traumatic event. The impact of trauma is greater for sensitives than for those not in that category. Think back to children you know or have known and how they look and respond to various experiences. See if you can identify those that might be sensitives. Perhaps you are one who is a sensitive soul and maybe this is the first validation you have received of that. Give it some consideration and see what you come up with. No wonder it is difficult to understand and make meaning out of PTSD, let alone write with clarity about it.

When someone experiences an actual threat to their life, body or some part of their body, it is usually both shocking and frightening to them and qualifies as trauma. Some examples might include: having your arm get mangled in a piece of machinery; being a civilian caught in a war zone; or, being a female soldier trapped and raped by a superior officer. It could be a single event or multiple events over time and when the experience is overwhelming, it qualifies as traumatic. Put simply, when such an event takes place, the psyche is overwhelmed and unable to function normally. There is not even agreement on what psyche is. I have seen it described as soul, spirit, personality, center of thought and feeling. Psyche is our soul or being, our Self with a capital S. Our personality, or sense of self with a small s, includes thoughts and feelings. For this discussion on PTSD, let us agree that psyche means our personal ability to think and act coherently.

When professionals first got together to categorize, describe and label what we now refer to as PTSD, they perceived PTSD as a weakness within the person who showed symptoms and they named it "traumatic neurosis." It meant that something was wrong with that person. During WWI they called it "shell shock" for a while and then "war neurosis." In WWII they began to call it "Battle Fatigue" and "Combat Stress Reaction" also known as CSR. In 1980, when professionals attempted again to describe what I am calling PTSD, they realized that it was more about the traumatic event and a person's response to it, than some inherent weakness or problem within them. To begin with, they thought of the traumatic event as a catastrophic stressor that was outside the range of usual human experience: meaning torture, war, rape, and disasters. They discovered that trauma cannot be objectified, any more than emotional pain can be, and that traumatic events come through each person's perception, perspective, and the meanings they give to the experience.

In 1994, when revisions to the Diagnostic and Statistical Manual took place, the criteria for PTSD included (1) a history of exposure to a traumatic event and symptoms from each of three symptom clusters: (2) intrusive recollections, (3) avoidant/numbing symptoms, and (4) hyper-arousal symptoms. A fifth criterion concerned duration of symptoms; and, a sixth stipulated that PTSD symptoms must cause significant distress or functional impairment. More recently, professionals agree that witnessing or even learning of a traumatic event, can lead to PTSD: specifically, learning that a loved one experienced a violent or accidental death or sexual violence in the form of rape.

Here are the latest definitions of Post-Traumatic Stress Disorder:

From the VA:
PTSD (post-traumatic stress disorder) is a mental health problem that some people develop after experiencing or witnessing a life-threatening event, like combat, a natural disaster, a car accident, or sexual assault.

From the Mayo Clinic:
Post-traumatic stress disorder (PTSD) is a mental health condition that is triggered by a terrifying event — either experiencing it or witnessing it. Symptoms may include flashbacks, nightmares and severe anxiety, as well as uncontrollable thoughts about the event.

From the American Psychiatric Association:

Post-traumatic stress disorder (PTSD) is a psychiatric disorder that can occur in people who have experienced or witnessed a traumatic event such as a natural disaster, a serious accident, a terrorist act, war/combat, rape or other violent personal assault. PTSD is a real illness that causes real suffering.

Anyone who has or is experiencing PTSD knows that last statement to be true. It is also more common than previously known. Recent data shows about four of every 100 American men (or 4%) and ten out every 100 American women (or 10%) will be diagnosed with PTSD in their lifetime. Even more reason for professionals and lay people alike to understand what PTSD is, how it can manifest in people's lives, and what can be done about it.

Here is the actual verbiage in the DSM V, (The Diagnostic and Statistical Manual of Mental Disorders, Fifth Edition) that professionals and insurance companies use to certify a diagnosis of PTSD. Read through this and then I will break it down.

**Criterion A (one required):** The person was exposed to: death, threatened death, actual or threatened serious injury, or actual or threatened sexual violence, in the following way(s):
- Direct exposure
- Witnessing the trauma
- Learning that a relative or close friend was exposed to a trauma
- Indirect exposure to aversive details of the trauma, usually in the course of professional duties (e.g., first responders, medics)

**Criterion B (one required):** The traumatic event is persistently re-experienced, in the following way(s):
- Intrusive thoughts
- Nightmares
- Flashbacks
- Emotional distress after exposure to traumatic reminders
- Physical reactivity after exposure to traumatic reminders

**Criterion C (one required):** Avoidance of trauma-related stimuli after the trauma, in the following way(s):
- Trauma-related thoughts or feelings
- Trauma-related reminders

**Criterion D (two required):** Negative thoughts or feelings that began or worsened after the trauma, in the following way(s):
- Inability to recall key features of the trauma
- Overly negative thoughts and assumptions about oneself or the world
- Exaggerated blame of self or others for causing the trauma
- Negative affect
- Decreased interest in activities
- Feeling isolated
- Difficulty experiencing positive affect

**Criterion E (two required):** Trauma-related arousal and reactivity that began or worsened after the trauma, in the following way(s):
- Irritability or aggression
- Risky or destructive behavior
- Hypervigilance
- Heightened startle reaction
- Difficulty concentrating
- Difficulty sleeping

**Criterion F (required):** Symptoms last for more than one month.

**Criterion G (required):** Symptoms create distress or functional impairment (e.g., social, occupational).

**Criterion H (required):** Symptoms are not due to medication, substance use, or other illness.

**Two specifications**:
- **Dissociative Specification.** In addition to meeting criteria for diagnosis, an individual experiences high levels of either of the following in reaction to trauma-related stimuli:
- **Depersonalization:** experience of being an outside observer of or detached from oneself (e.g., feeling as if "this is not happening to me" or one were in a dream).
- **Derealization:** experience of unreality, distance, or distortion (e.g., "things are not real").
- **Delayed Specification.** Full diagnostic criteria are not met until at least six months after the trauma(s), although onset of symptoms may occur immediately.

Let's break down some of what was described above starting with intrusive recollections. These can be actual memories with all the sensory information (sights, sounds, smells, sensations, tastes), or it can be an image, picture of some part of your past trauma, or an intrusive thought or belief related to yourself or the trauma. These intrusive recollections come to you unbidden. In other words, you did nothing to bring this on. We do not know what the many potential triggers are that can bring on traumatic memories/intrusive recollections of any kind. It could be something you see or hear in your neighborhood, on the TV, while walking, on a trip somewhere or even in your dreams. For me, it is often the sound of a helicopter that triggers my memories and body reactions. Once, I was walking from my car in the parking lot to the store when two things happened simultaneously that caused a severe reaction. The two things were, a siren from an ambulance going by and the sound of a helicopter overhead. I was immediately triggered. My mind knew where I was but my body was sure I was back in Vietnam with casualties coming in during an attack on our base camp.

One time about sixteen years ago, I was in aikido training and the back door was open. I had never been in the dojo with that door open before. I felt the summer heat from outside and started to experience some smells that automatically took me back to Vietnam. I went to the back of the dojo, looked out the back door and what I saw was a street in Vietnam, even though I was actually in West Seattle. I use these examples to help you understand what triggers can be and the effects they can have. If someone would have told me that having the back door of the aikido dojo open could produce that response in me, I would not have believed that possible.

Now let us check out flashbacks. Triggers can bring on flashbacks. When we are in a flashback, we do not know where we are. The flashback tells us we are in another place and time. The example I gave you above of seeing the street in Vietnam, was a flashback. Here is another example, and one of my worst. I was driving to work on the freeway when I saw an actual OD green army truck. Seeing the truck was the trigger that brought on the flashback. Next, I saw a similar army truck filled with soldiers. The soldiers had dirty faces, like those in the Vietnam War, and many were bandaged with blood all over their faces, arms and uniforms. The most painful part of the flashback was the pleading eyes of the soldiers who seemed to be dying. I did not know what was happening to me at the time because I had not yet been diagnosed with PTSD. Even though it was 1978 and eleven years after my return from Vietnam, and I had never had a flashback. Remember I was driving at the time. I did what many of you have done; I held my breath while that was happening. My body started to shake and I realized somewhere inside me that I was in trouble and better pull over. It is a miracle that I was able to safely pull over to the side of the road where I stopped while my body acted as though it was having a convulsion. I shook and shook all over and cried and cried aloud, "What is happening to me?" That was the experience that led me to seek help. Flashbacks are powerful experiences that are probably the most telling sign that we have lived through trauma.

If you look at Criterion B's list, you will see emotional and physical reactivity after a traumatic reminder. My crying and shaking after that flashback, is an example of both of those. Crying is an emotional release and shaking is a physiological release. Peter Levine Ph.D. describes what animals do when they have a harrowing experience that is life threatening. They lie down and let their whole body shake until all the terror is released from their body. We humans have a cerebral cortex which limits what we allow our bodies to do, so most people will not lay their body down after a trauma and allow it to shake it out.

Looking back at the list of criteria for diagnosis, the only other one I believe might need some further clarification is hypervigilance. My guess is that if you have PTSD, you know what that is, but to be clear for all readers, it is always looking all around everywhere for potential danger lurking. It might be scanning the room, environment, looking out the sides of your eyes as well as forward. Instead of being vigilant or cautious, you are super alert for the slightest indication of an attack from anywhere and it often includes looking for the paths to any exits, ensuring that you have a clear path out of any situation. It means being keenly watchful and ready to respond. This comes under Criterion E, which used to be referred to as hyper-arousal and includes: heightened anxiety and vigilance, having trouble falling asleep and/or staying asleep, being irritable and even angry. Judith Herman M.D., the author of the book *Trauma and Recovery,* refers to hyper-arousal as the first cardinal symptom of PTSD and states that the "traumatized person startles easily, reacts irritably to small provocations, and sleeps poorly." (Page 35) All of these symptoms come from the chronic arousal of the autonomic nervous system, which will be discussed further in the chapter on the body and the brain.

All that said, you could look, sound and behave normally but also have PTSD. When you are in the throes of the condition and symptoms, you would not look or sound normal. You might feel on edge, avoid people and places that remind you of the trauma, have nightmares, jump at sudden noises, be wary all the time and stay home rather than go out and deal with people and places, and of course, have flashbacks. You might be very irritable and angry, such that any small response from someone could set you off into a tirade completely disproportionate to his or her response. You could feel emotionally cut off from others, feeling numb, depressed, anxious, having trouble concentrating or sleeping. You may even fear the of loss of control and thus need to control everything around you. These are some of the most telling signs of PTSD. During the traumatic event(s) a person may feel their life, and even the lives of others, are in danger, leaving them with a feeling of helplessness. If people do get hurt, it is common to feel guilty that you did not do something to stop it, even though you were unable to help. Once past the trauma, it follows you into the PTSD so that you may feel the need to control everything, in order never to be in that situation again where you felt and were helpless, people were hurt because you did not DO something to save or protect them.

At the heart of PTSD is the inability to stay present in the moment. When the trauma is so ever present that you seem to live there, more than in the present, and you are constantly hyper-vigilant, on edge, irritable, anxious, scanning for anything unexpected and unwanted that could bring harm, having nightmares and flashbacks, feeling alone, isolated, and unable to feel connected to your loved ones or yourself, you cannot *be in the moment,* and connected to your physical body sensations. That inability is the main sign that you have PTSD and it is also the remedy. Learning to be connected to yourself, your body and body sensations, and to stay present in the moment, helps you detach and heal from the PTSD. At the time of the trauma, staying present in your body and in the moment was the last thing you wanted — in fact, getting away and out of your body was your goal, but due to the circumstances of the traumatic situation, you could not. Untreated trauma means that you were not able to return to your normal functioning and stayed stuck in avoidance of anything remotely like the traumatic situation, therefore, not present in your body and the moment.

During a disaster or traumatic event when you are helpless to do anything worthwhile to change what is happening, you feel utter powerlessness and either freeze, explode emotionally or do meaningless actions in relation to what is needed. When frozen, you are not able to respond in any way and are out of touch with yourself. When exploding, emotionally the same is true. You are being driven by your raging response to your helplessness. The meaningless actions could be picking up small pieces of glass after an explosion or firefight. None of those are effective actions in relation to the traumatic experience, but are survival mechanisms that helped you get through what you were experiencing. Once on the other side of the trauma, it is important to return to your normal functioning. In the military that is unlikely, as you are still required to go on with your mission and your unit. Using my own experiences again, when we were being mortared and I was scrubbed in as an operating room nurse, it was my duty to stay standing and do my job handing instruments to the surgeon. I know that I did that and did that well, even when I was somewhat numb. I suspect for many soldiers in the midst of a firefight, they kept going even when their buddies were being blown up beside them. They kept going but were likely somewhat frozen/numb "steeled against the worst emotional response." Basically, for each of us, we could not allow our emotional responses to what was happening to break through, so we literally "steeled ourselves against it," blocked and blunted our ability to sense and feel our emotions. Then the task months or years later was to undo the "steel" or "freeze."

The following came from an interview with Erin Findley Ph.D., a medical anthropologist and the author of the book, *Fields of Combat: Understanding PTSD among Veterans of Iraq and Afghanistan*. "For many years, much of what was widely understood about PTSD – our cultural ideas about PTSD – was influenced by the fact that the clinical and research communities had not yet developed the scientific knowledge to understand what causes PTSD, how it works within the body and the mind, and how best to treat it. As a result, PTSD was thought of as a chronic and disabling illness for which there was no cure."

Note the past tense, *was thought of* as chronic and disabling — not so anymore. I'm happy to see a professional agreeing with my belief that PTSD can be healed to the point that people who experience it can go on to live normal lives, free of everyday symptoms of PTSD. That does not mean they never get triggered; it does mean they can handle triggering responses which are limited in number and intensity. It does mean focused therapy is necessary to work though the trauma and develop resources to deal with any triggering experiences.

Erin Findley did many interviews with both male and female veterans for her research and ended up with a complex kaleidoscope of PTSD, which showed her "there is no one way of viewing or experiencing post-traumatic stress. The task then became how to convey that complexity to the reader, and the best way seemed to be to let veterans and other participants speak for themselves as much as possible."

# Chapter 9
# OUR BODY, BRAIN, AND PTSD

During the years from 1985-2019, I was doing trauma resolution therapy as a nurse psychotherapist and attended many symposiums and workshops lead by Dr. Bessel Van Der Kolk. In more recent years, I read and reread his book: *The Body Keeps the Score*. I was heavily influenced by his work and the work of Dr. Judith Herman, the author of the book, *Trauma and Recovery*, which will be evident in much of what follows.

One terrifying moment has the power to alter your mind and body. Trauma causes actual physiological changes in the brain and nervous system, including how the brain's alarm systems work, increases in the release of stress hormones, and the identification and categorization of important and irrelevant information. Research has shown that the signals we receive in our body that tell us we are alive, do not work very well during and after trauma.

When we are born, our brain is still developing. The part of our brain that helps us as babies is referred to as the reptilian brain. It is located in our brain stem at the top of our spine, which is the lowest part of our actual brain. On top of that brain stem is the hypothalamus. Those two parts work together to control the energy levels of the body and the functioning of the heart, lungs, endocrine and immune systems. Above the brain stem is the limbic system which includes the amygdala, the hypothalamus, and hippocampus and the medial and prefrontal cortex. The limbic system is also known as the mammalian brain and is the seat of our emotions, the monitor of threats and what is pleasurable or not, important and not. (For reference see picture page 139)

The top layer of the brain is our neocortex or thinking brain. Here we can plan, reflect, imagine, speak and write, rather than act out what we feel. This part of our brain is nonfunctional during trauma and when triggered.

If we cannot run, hide, get away, or fight because we are being held down, trapped, thwarted or blocked in some way — the chemicals inside us are still secreting hormones and the electrical circuits are still firing and we become agitated, aroused or collapse.

In PTSD, when there is a release of stress hormones, it has been shown that those stress hormones remain elevated even after the traumatic event has ended. The amygdala in the person with PTSD perceives the threat as still there, ongoing. This was shown in Van Der Kolk's neuroimaging studies on brains of patients with PTSD.

Those neuroimaging studies of people with PTSD reported by Dr. Bessel Van Der Kolk also show that when someone is having intense fear, grief, or anger, the amygdala is activated while the medial frontal area of the brain is either not functioning well or is shut down. That person may seem to behave erratically, doing things that do not make sense, responding out of proportion to what others perceive as happening. For example, a woman who was sexually assaulted in the military may respond to a gentle, compassionate touch as though it is an assault.

Because of trauma, the executive functioning of the medial prefrontal cortex of our brain is rendered offline; its function is literally taken over by the loud expressiveness of the amygdala and the limbic system. The emotional brain is in charge, rather than the rational brain, and the trauma survivor is emotionally out of control, angrily blowing up at both little and big issues. The medial prefrontal cortex is unable to regulate emotions and that is cause for serious problems, especially in relationships, because the person with PTSD is unable to be rational in any way when the amygdala is in charge. "When the alarm bell of the emotional brain keeps signaling that you are in danger, no amount of insight will silence it." (*Body Keeps the Score*, page 64)

A significant finding from this research is that a person with PTSD often cannot verbalize their experience, as the Broca's Area – the brain's speech center – goes "offline" during the trauma or triggering event, essentially not functioning. A trigger or triggering event is anything that reminds you of the trauma or traumatic event and produces an emotional and/or physiological response commensurate with the actual trauma. You can fully experience the trauma, terror, rage, helplessness, and the impulse to fight/flight/freeze but not be able to put it into words. This finding is particularly helpful for both civilian and military police to know, since they often discount a trauma survivor's authenticity and believability when the survivor cannot articulate clearly, in sequence, all the aspects of the traumatic event on command. The pressure from police to give the details of the experience and show emotion is an added trauma to survivors. I firmly believe all police, both civilian and military, need to be educated in dealing with people who have experienced a traumatic event and how to elicit the information they need. Police need to understand how survivors respond to trauma and be both patient and compassionate.

Another important finding in Van Der Kolk's research is that the right side of the brain is activated in those with PTSD and the left side deactivated. The right side is intuitive, visual, spatial and emotional, plus stores sensual memories of sound, smells, and touch. The left side is analytical, linguistic and sequential, remembers facts, statistics and has vocabulary. Van Der Kolk's research identifies that the right side of the brain in someone with PTSD reacts automatically to voices, facial features and gestures from the past. Because the left brain is deactivated in trauma, someone with PTSD would likely be unable to report the logical sequence of the traumatic experience and put that experience into coherent words. Trauma survivors often report, "losing their minds," which is akin to not being able to think logically or speak coherently about their experience in any logical sequential manner. The latter is problematic when there is a report made to the police, whether civilian or military. When something reminds the survivor of the past trauma, they re-experience it as though it is happening to them in the moment and they are helpless. Brain scans show that such a person cannot be present in the moment they are living, but rather are stuck in the past trauma. They are not living fully and not fully experiencing themselves or life. They cannot integrate new experiences and can't grow as a person until they deal with the trauma and develop new internal resources. One way of thinking about it is, that the trauma survivor is frozen in their past.

It is as though they have a different nervous system focused on suppressing the inner chaos and stress. Those added stress hormones can lead to debilitating physiological conditions such as fibromyalgia, chronic fatigue syndrome and other auto immune diseases. Once activated, the brain's alarm system is programmed to find escape through running, stop and fight, or freeze in place. We do these things automatically until we come to our senses and become aware of the current reality. I experienced this in my own life back in January of 1968, when I was returning from a year in Vietnam.

I was in Los Angeles to visit nursing friends I had worked with before going to Vietnam. My friend Ellie was driving me to the hospital where I had worked and suddenly there was an ambulance with a siren blaring. My automatic response was to dive into the footwell of the car. Once down there my mind clicked on, and I realized what I had done automatically. Ellie was looking at me and said, "What are you doing?" My amygdala decided based on the siren, that I was in potential danger and sent me diving into the footwell of the car. Once there, the prefrontal cortex part of my brain came back online and I became aware of the siren. This allowed me to realize that I was no longer in the war zone and I sheepishly sat back in my seat. Only twenty-four hours earlier I was in the war zone. The amygdala's danger signal sent cortisol and adrenalin into my body which increased my blood pressure, breathing and heart rate so I could respond to the potential threat. This same type of reaction can happen years later. I described my reaction to a trigger earlier with the ambulance and helicopter.

Our hippocampus is a lot like our computer's memory that writes files to its hard drive. After a trauma, our hippocampus works to remember the event accurately and make sense of it, but because a trauma is typically overwhelming, all the information does not get coded correctly. This means that we might have trouble remembering important details of the event, or we might find ourselves thinking a lot about what happened because our hippocampus is working so hard to try to make sense of things.

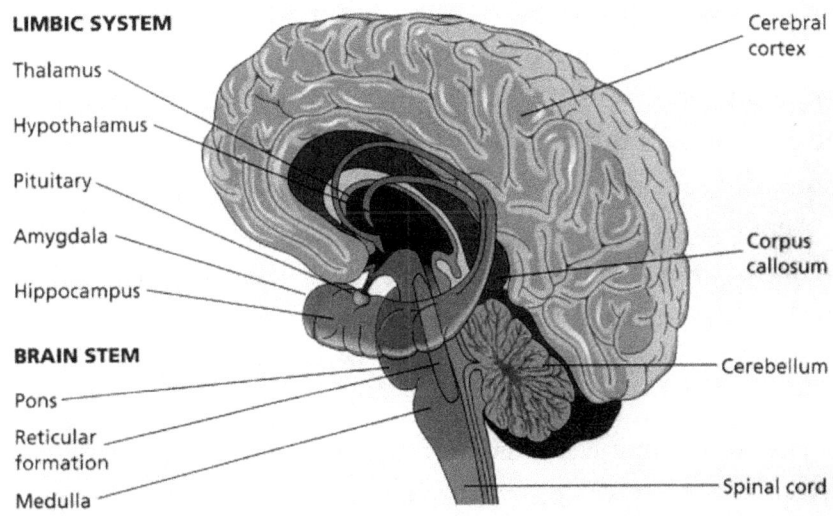

26. Image from class I took on Interpersonal Neurobiology about 28 years ago. This shows the brain stem and the limbic system with parts named. I have not been able to find original source. It is a teaching tool.

As stated previously, the limbic system comprises the thalamus, hypothalamus, hippocampus, amygdala, and connecting pathways. It mediates and expresses emotional, motivational, sexual and social behaviors and memory. The brain absorbs information from the outside world, interprets it, and makes the body act accordingly. It does this through a fascinating process of communication between specialized brain or neural cells – called neurons – that fire electrical impulses, or thoughts. The largest web of neocortical functioning in the brain is between the prefrontal area and the limbic structures. This perhaps explains the great variety of emotions that humans experience. The amygdala plays a large role in processing emotions.

The key to creating emotional health is putting a gap between an event and our response. When impulse happens, usually from the amygdala (the fear center of the brain), meaning is formed through appraisal. It is in the gap that the trigger – the conditioned response – occurs and you experience the response in your body. For example, your first experience on a Ferris wheel may be exhilarating or terrifying. The memory will be stored as such, and will be recalled at any time the word Ferris wheel is mentioned. In this way you form emotional habits. The good news is that cognitive reframing allows you to change your emotional habits to enjoy a life of more ease!

Appraisal of the level of threat, through the operation of the thalamus, hypothalamus, and limbic system, is the trigger for an emotional response. Appraisal is a source of autonomic (involuntary) arousal; the emotional response is mediated by the autonomic nervous system.

The Autonomic Nervous System (ANS) is part of the peripheral nervous system. It is a collection of neurons that influence the activity of many different organs, including the stomach, heart, and lungs. Within the ANS, there are two subsystems that have mostly opposing effects:

- **The sympathetic nervous system (SNS):** Neurons within the SNS generally prepare the body to react to something in its environment, such as increase heart rate to prepare a person to escape from danger.
- **The parasympathetic nervous system (PNS):** Parasympathetic neurons mostly regulate bodily functions when a person is at rest.

- One critical function of the ANS is to prepare the body for action through the "fight or flight" response. It moves blood to muscles so you can fight or flee. If the body perceives a threat in the environment, the sympathetic neurons of the ANS react by: increasing heart rate widening the airways to make breathing easier releasing stored energy increasing strength in the muscles slowing digestion and other bodily processes that are less important for action

These changes prepare the body to respond appropriately to a threat in the environment. (Medical News Today.com January 10, 2020)

In a normal situation, when the threat or perceived threat ceases, the parasympathetic nervous system shifts the body into restorative mode, which reduces stress hormones, decreases heart rate, relaxes muscles, restores normal breathing and allows the brain to shift back to the normal top-down structure. For those twenty percent of trauma survivors who go on to develop symptoms of post-traumatic stress disorder, the shift from reactive to restorative mode never occurs and the emotional brain stays in charge. The emotional brain continues to produce sensations that lead to the PTSD sufferer feeling scared and unable to help themselves.

Scientific research shows that after trauma your brain goes through biological changes that it wouldn't have experienced if there had been no trauma. The impact of these changes is especially exacerbated by three major brain function dysregulations:

- **Overstimulated amygdala:** The amygdala is responsible for alerting you to potential threat, plus tagging memories with emotion. After a trauma the amygdala can stay on high alert and is in an activated loop during which it looks for and perceives threat everywhere.
- **Underactive hippocampus:** An increase in the stress hormone glucocorticoid which kills cells in the hippocampus, and renders it less effective in making synaptic connections necessary for memory consolidation. This situation keeps both the body and mind stimulated in reactive mode or high arousal.
- **Ineffective variability:** The constant elevation of stress hormones interferes with the body's ability to regulate itself. The sympathetic nervous system continues to be highly activated which

leads to fatigue of the body and several of its systems, especially the adrenals. (*The Science Behind PTSD Symptoms: How Trauma Changes The Brain*, by Michele Rosenthal June 27, 2019)

One of the worst aspects of trauma is the feeling that it is never ending. My favorite descriptive phrase for it is, "the gift that goes on giving." Those who have experienced trauma know that there seem to be endless triggers to flashbacks and they can show up anytime. When the trauma is unhealed, it can feel as if the triggers are endless and always intense. Once you go through the healing process and have discharged most of the energy from the trauma, the triggers are milder and infrequent. They are also easier to handle because you have so many more tools to deal with them, you are clearer and stronger and because of that, those triggers have less power. You have more power over yourself and your responses to the triggers.

During the actual original traumatic event, it is common for the person experiencing the trauma to split off emotions and sensations, sights, sounds, images and thoughts because it is so overwhelming. Those aspects of the trauma that are split off are readily available to return and harass you as flashbacks, if they are not reconnected to you. It is through therapy that all parts of the trauma are reconnected and integrated. In therapy, all the parts of the puzzle are put together through the extensive work you do with your therapist. In the process, you learn to identify your bodily sensations and emotions, name them, and know that you are safe, even as you allow yourself to experience them gradually with more and more intensity. Through therapy, you learn to stay grounded in the present moment and reconnect to all of you, including those emotions and sensations that were previously split off in the trauma. You will bring back all that was split off during the trauma and you become more whole. Learning to stay present in the moment and in your body is essential to your healing. To do that you need to know and feel that you are safe, and it can be a long process to get to that point. I have seen cases where it took years for the person to feel safe enough to go deep enough to heal the trauma, but once there it can go relatively fast. It is easy to see that a trusting relationship with your therapist is critical to feeling safe.

Those who respond to their trauma by freezing are numb, unfeeling and their mind is blank. They shut everything down. If you took a picture of them in that state, the picture would show them in a blank stare as though no one is home. They are not thinking, feeling, remembering or understanding what they are experiencing. It is easy to see that this person could not give any information about their trauma to anyone asking, including a therapist or investigator. Working with their breathing, heart rate, body movement, dancing, drumming and two other tools we will focus on later – EFT (Emotional Freedom Technique) and EMDR (Eye Movement Desensitization Reprocessing) – will help them be present in their body and begin to feel again.

Imagine you are walking through a park when out of nowhere the man in front of you gets smacked by an errant Frisbee. Automatically, you recoil in sympathy. Or you're watching a race, and you feel your own heart racing with excitement as the runners vie to cross the finish line first. Or you see a woman sniff some unfamiliar food and wrinkle her nose in disgust. Suddenly, your own stomach turns at the thought of the meal. How do we understand, so immediately and instinctively, their thoughts, feelings and intentions? Mirror neurons are a type of brain cell that respond equally when we perform an action and when we witness someone else perform the same action. It is through these mirror neurons that we develop empathy.

Often a major problem with trauma that makes it difficult to talk about and overcome, is when the survivor is carrying shame. It could be shame about something they did or had done to them or the way they responded or did not. When someone feels shame, it is difficult to look another person in the eyes and be close or intimate with them. Often these people hate or despise themselves for what happened to them, or how they perceive themselves based on their reactions at the time of the trauma.

# Chapter 10
# ESSENTIALS OF TREATMENT

If you are not a therapist reading this chapter, be aware that some of the words are directed toward the therapist, yet intended to educate everyone as to what is essential in order for therapy to be successful. Use this as a guide so that if your therapist is not following these essentials, you can have a conversation with them and let them know what you need. Many of the words are directed to you, the trauma survivor, to help you heal from your trauma.

First and foremost in treatment is you, the therapist, being authentically you, open hearted and listening deeply. Listen for what is said and not said. Listen for feelings not expressed, listen inside yourself for what you are experiencing. You are the medicine! I once gave a workshop to professionals on behalf of the Department of Veterans Affairs in Washington State and titled it: YOU ARE THE MEDICINE. Most of the trauma you will be dealing with happened in relationship to someone: a family, a military unit, a predator, a group, therefore, it must be healed in a relationship. You are it!

In order for your client/patient to trust you, you must be trustworthy. What you say must be truthful. You will need to be congruent. That means your facial expressions must match what you are saying. If your face shows disgust at something your client/patient has described to you and you deny what you are feeling/experiencing, they will not trust you. Keep in mind that many of your client's/patient's families did not validate what was perceived accurately by the person you are working with. More than anything, each person needs their accurate perceptions validated. If you are being less than truthful or try to cover up what you are feeling/experiencing, they will know. In the beginning, they may not be empowered enough to confront you but the damage to the relationship will already be done.

Your success and their healing depend on how much of you, the therapist, is present and available to them — NOT any specific method or technique you know or apply. If you have had a stressful week, are sitting in your office with a veteran or trauma survivor diagnosed with PTSD, and your mind is on an interaction you had with your co-worker at lunch, you are not being fully present or authentic. The veteran in the chair will know and feel that you are not present with them. They may feel unimportant and discounted by you. They need you to be fully engaged with them no matter what. Being fully present with them means that your focus, mind and heart are all right there in the moment with the veteran or trauma survivor across from you.

Have you ever been with a therapist who was responding to you from their head and not their heart? It is one thing to be in a professional seminar and hear therapists speaking from their head because they are discussing a specific topic, but totally another to be with that therapist when you are seeking relief from emotional distress and instead of being with you and your feelings, they are in their head. When that happens, you cannot feel the connection with them because they are not connecting with you. We humans connect with our hearts, not our heads. It is tempting to stay in your head if what you are faced with is difficult, yet that is the least therapeutic thing you can do. Challenging as it is, if you chose to be a psychotherapist/psychologist or psychiatrist/mental health counselor, you need to commit to being fully yourself, open hearted and available emotionally to those you choose to serve.

If you have someone in your office who is clearly in emotional distress, what do you have to give him or her? You have you, your heart, a human connection, your listening skills, and all that you know about responding and dealing with someone in that level of distress. If you are only offering them what you know, rather than the YOU that knows, how successful do you believe you will be?

It is not easy to be a therapist and it is especially not easy to work with veterans and others with severe trauma. If you have chosen that path, I thank you sincerely. Our veterans need you and so do many others with painful traumas to heal. Thank you for your dedication, and putting yourself on the line to do this very important work. It is not easy to hear the many descriptions of traumatic events, see the effects in your clients/patients, then reach into your toolkit to offer comfort and peace to them, as well as lead them out. They will need to dip into their trauma at times and then come back out. The further into therapy they go, the deeper into the actual trauma they can go. The key is to come fully out of it before the end of the session. Your job as therapist is to stay with them wherever they go.

When I was actively doing the work myself, I often had to jump in the foxhole, pipe, explosion, sinking boat, with them. In order to be fully present with a trauma survivor while they are reliving the trauma, it is often necessary to be at their side as they delve into the depths of their traumatic event. I remember an EMT (Emergency Medical Technician) I worked with years ago who had trauma from age three and who would hide inside a large empty pipe. I had to go into the pipe with him energetically and sit with him to connect, until he could talk with me. With veterans, think of it as going into the foxhole, trench, alley, with them. You may not have to say much. Simply be there and let them know, "I am here with you and I will stay here until you feel safe enough to tell me what you are experiencing." It is up to you to determine, with your skills, how much is enough at the time. It may be how much you can handle or how much you perceive the veteran/client can handle. At some point, if it does not happen naturally, you need to bring them out. If previously, you and your client created a safe place to be, you can move them from where they are to that safe place. If you did not already create a safe place, then draw them to where you are, in the here and now. Examples: "Their name, let that go for now and gently bring your focus back to (that safe place we have used before) the office/group room and be with me/us here." To create a safe place, have the client in their imagination create one either outdoors or indoors. An example of an outdoor safe place could be on a secluded private beach in the tropics, or a private mountain retreat described as they choose. An indoor place might be a room in a house that the client owns and designed/decorated as they choose. You can ask them "if you could have the best or most perfect safe place to go to when you are feeling triggered, depressed, or fearful what would it look like and where would it be? The key is for them to designate where it is and what it looks and feels like.

At some level, each trauma survivor wants to know from you if you have what it takes to stay with them through the worst of their experiences and feelings. It is as though they test you. "If I tell you this gory graphic story, will you hear me and not disappear or go away inside yourself? Will you stay with me through it all?" Veterans especially might do that. They know the horrors they saw, heard, felt and no one ever wants to hear all the details, yet telling the details and remembering when they are ready, is essential. Consider what they may be carrying inside themselves and have been carrying for years. Can you, as a therapist, listen, stay present, feel your own feelings and hold the veteran and the story while they reveal it to you? This is not the starting place but it is a place you both need to get to for the healing to take place. As the therapist, you need to be ready for whatever the veteran needs to release. All releases need to be done in safe, healthy ways for both of you.

In the beginning, offer different ways for the veteran or trauma survivor to release anger. I always had a large, ugly, strong pillow and tennis rackets available to pound on and yell with and a large punching pad and punching gloves, plus heavy durable towels to twist. It is helpful to have things like that available. I worked in the basement of my home which I bought specifically for therapy. I had a separate office and outside the office was a large group room with tennis rackets, pillows, a large anger pad, a counter top with clay and people toys to manipulate and use to tell stories. I also had puppets, shelves with figurines of all different types that could be used for sand-tray work, sheets of different types and sizes, blankets, and ropes. I had whatever I thought could be a helpful tool to assist clients in releasing their stories and trauma. Many of the items I had were used for child work and even baby work for those with early trauma and for different types of psychodrama work.

I began one-on-one with each person to get to know them and build trust. I did not take people into their worst trauma until after I had been working with them for over a year and knew what inner resources they had and that our relationship was solid. I often would work with them for about three or four months individually and then put them in a group. My groups were not like normal group therapy. I did individual therapy with each person within the group setting. I gave each person a group manual that included guidelines, structures we use in group, self-care contracts, ground rules and a lot of specific information they could use during their therapy. The group became like a healthy family to support each person doing the therapeutic work they needed to do. There were from six to nine people in the groups. What I found very interesting and miraculous, was that everyone in the group came from an unhealthy family and none of them had healthy communication skills, yet in the group they spoke and behaved as though they grew up in a healthy family, had healthy communication skills and utilized them well. The culture in the group encouraged each member to be their best self and to call out the best in each other and hold each other accountable to their contracts. They did that and modeled for each other. Each person had both self-care contracts and personal contracts they created. (See appendix page 231)

Whether in the individual session or in group, each person was in charge of their own agenda. They either came prepared with something they wanted to change, work through, release, or something would come up in the session organically. In the group, anyone could be triggered at any time. That is one of the values of working in a group setting. One person might be enacting a psychodrama of a traumatic moment in their family when another person watching or playing a role in the psychodrama is triggered and remembers their own trauma. During the time when everyone is processing the just completed work, they can speak up about their own trigger(s) and potentially work through it by doing their own therapeutic work. Another value of working within a group/healthy family is that you have a support system that is ongoing and you can call one another to check out clear/unclear thinking, share a trigger and how you worked through it, ask for affirmations, or validation of a perception. Because of the structure of group and rules of confidentiality it is safe to do that with other group members.

Earlier, I described to you a day in which I was driving and encountered a white truck on the freeway. That is a classic example of me being triggered, and me showing up at my therapist's office/group room in the midst of it. It took about thirty minutes for my body to calm down and me be able to talk without sounding strident. I do not remember what Elaine said or did but I do remember telling her what I saw, felt, heard, and what it connected to in my Vietnam experiences. I do remember she was fully present with me and listening fully and I could feel her empathic responses to what I was experiencing and her desire to help me get through it to the other side and feel calm again. I do remember that she did not use any particular technique that I am aware of, but rather she was with me, supporting and encouraging me to describe the trigger and the source of it in my Vietnam experiences. Before the session was over, I was feeling more myself and very grateful to have her there with me and helping me.

Triggers can be frightening because they are so sudden and you feel like you and your life, in that moment, are totally out of control. It takes every ounce of intention and desire to get back to being who you are and not feeling overwhelmed.

It is helpful to know what some of your triggers are, and most trauma survivors do know some of them and do their best to avoid those triggering places or experiences. I am not sure it is possible to know all the triggers and avoid them, or even if that is desirable. I believe that being triggered is helpful in working through the trauma and the more you can work through the trauma, the less power it has over you. In the group setting, because there are many potential triggers, each person has many opportunities in that supportive environment to work through aspects of their trauma and ultimately all of it. That said, if you are new to therapy or not in therapy, you are likely to be triggered and not have the tools and therapeutic support to work them through. It is important to find someone to help you. Someone who has the skills and background to help you heal from your trauma.

If you are a veteran, there are many local, state and federal clinics where you can access help. The Veteran's Administration has hospitals and clinics in many areas. The various State Department of Veterans Affairs have access to resources for therapy as do many counties. Call or look them up online. For civilians, do a search for a therapist who specifically works with trauma survivors and when you have a list, call them and ask for a free twenty-minute interview with them. See how it feels to be with them, ask them how they work with trauma survivors, see if you can feel them and their heart while with them, ask them how they would handle it if you showed up triggered. Ask them if they can handle (whatever you believe the worst of your trauma is, e.g., rape) if you were describing it to them, and any other questions you have.

You are not your trauma, but if you were traumatized and the trauma is activated in you, it may seem like you have lost the true you, the empowered you. The trauma is so loud in your life that there is no space for you and who you really are. Think about that for a moment. Do you know who you are at the deepest level? Do you like who you are? Did you get lost along the way and lose touch with who you truly are? Did your pain from your trauma take over your life so that is all you focus on? Did your behavior to deal with the pain of the trauma take over? Often trauma survivors begin to do things to lessen their pain and then get stuck or caught up in an addictive pattern that takes over their life. Addictive patterns can be with drugs, alcohol, food, sex, relationships, self-harm, avoidance, isolation, smoking, etc.

One of the biggest challenges with trauma resolution are addictions. If the survivor is addicted, they and you as therapist, must deal with the addiction first. It is impossible to do the deep healing work to resolve the trauma when someone is actively in an addiction. When the survivor relies on the addictive substance/behavior to avoid dealing with the trauma and associated feelings, there is no room for healing. The traumatized person cannot even approach dealing with the trauma until they are free of any and all addictions. Here is the operating principle: "You cannot heal what you cannot feel." That being the case, know that all addictions serve to cover feelings. The pattern of covering up or avoiding feelings has to be changed, decreased and eliminated in order to feel fully and heal.

When you believe you have big intense feelings that you have been avoiding or cannot access, it takes courage and determination to open up to feel them. It may also take ingenuity to come up with a way that works to access them. As an example, when looking back to my own story, I found it necessary to put up a wall around my heart to deal with all that I was seeing there at the 12$^{th}$ Evacuation Hospital at Cu Chi, Vietnam. Later, I had to strengthen that wall even more when I was at the University of Washington and learned about the fall of Saigon in 1975. That wall was so tall and so strong, it remained in place for me until I finally found a way to take it down. What happened was that when I was in therapy with Elaine, and I would reach in to find the feelings and would hit the wall. I focused on understanding how it worked. It took months, but eventually I discovered what seemed to be a metal corrugated door that would come down fast and hard between me and any feelings I had. Once I made that discovery, I had to come up with a way to stop that door. It was trial and error for a few weeks and finally with a lot of determination and focus, I decided to get a small stone and have it ready so I could slip it in under that door as it would slam down hard and fast to prevent me from having those feelings. I did that several times with stones of different sizes. Once I could get a bigger stone/rock under it, there was a space to work with. Next, I found a metal bar I could get under the door and create more space. By that time, the door was starting to get the message that it was no longer needed. I created a stronger longer metal rod to wedge under the metal corrugated door. There was enough space then for some feelings to start getting through. I continued to work at it and tell the door/wall that it was no longer needed because I was home, safe and wanted and needed to feel all of my feelings. I kept using the metal rod to push up the door more and more, plus talking to the door/wall and eventually it got the message and would not come slamming down to protect me from my feelings. Instead, I was in charge, and it was okay to have all my feelings and to learn how to deal with them. I did learn through the group process, and later in the training I went through for years, how to utilize the therapeutic process as a professional.

When I was ready, I began to work with Elaine as her assistant in some of her groups. Over time, as her clients grew to trust me, I did more and more therapy with them. I did that for years before I started my own groups. One key lesson for people and groups is on passivity.

It is about passive behavior and begins with discounting. What is it that people discount?

| **Yourself** | **Others** | **Situations** |
|---|---|---|
| Thoughts | Thoughts | What it is |
| Feelings | Feelings | Where it is |
| Wants | Wants | When it is |
| Needs | Needs | How it will be |
| Actions | Actions | Importance of it |

You may discount yourself more than others or others more than yourself. You may discount your thoughts, feelings, wants, needs, and be super-responsible about your actions. You may also discount others' actions especially toward you. You may discount everything about others or only some things. You may discount situations in many ways or only a few ways. Some people are always late, or come unprepared. Look through this list and see where you are on it. What fits you and is that okay with you now in your life? These are discounts — and discounting leads to passive behavior. Some of you may have been discounted in your life regularly, and know what it feels like. Your presence may have been discounted, not seen or heard, or responded to. It is painful. You may have had your feelings and needs discounted in your family. That too is painful. When you have been discounted regularly you learn to be passive.

**PASSIVE BEHAVIOR.** (+ means energy and it builds)
1. DO NOTHING - Ex: you are angry and do nothing about it,
+
2. OVERADAPT - Trying to please others and take care of others.
++
3. AGITATE - A variety of purposeless activities that do nothing to solve the problem.
+++ All addictions are a form of agitation. Some others are biting fingernails, playing with your hair on head or face, wiggling legs or feet. If someone in your office is wiggling/shaking their foot— gently put your hand on their foot and see what happens or ask them, "What is your leg saying right now?"
4. INCAPACITATE - Sending your energy inside so you get sick OR
++++
5. ESCALATE - Sending your energy outward by being violent or acting out in some way. ++++

INSTEAD OF BEING PASSIVE –BE ACCOUNTABLE FOR EVERYTHING IN YOUR LIFE.

If you, the survivor, are ready to do the deep healing work and you know you have an addiction, tell your therapist. The first step is stopping the addiction so you can be fully you and feel your feelings, in order to heal. You can join a twelve-step program to support you as you stop the addictive behavioral pattern. You can also begin the trust building in the therapy relationship. Every therapist that works with trauma survivors needs to know that touching the inner wounds in any way is very risky in someone working through an addiction. That is why I recommend not doing any therapy on the trauma at all until the survivor has at least one full year of consistent sobriety from whatever their addiction is. Some may need more than a year of solid sobriety before touching the traumatic material. When it comes to dealing directly with severe trauma, it is better to be safe than sorry and better to go slow. Start with a less intense trauma or only a small piece of the larger trauma.

As the therapist, you need to be observant of the client's breathing, posture, movements, changes in skin coloration, sweating, agitation, escalation, attempts at over-adaptation. Note these and anything else of importance, whether in individual session or in group sessions. These are indicators of what might be going on inside. Then you can say what you see and ask about it, for example: "I see that your shoulders are being held very stiffly, check in and tell me what you are aware of." "I noticed that your breathing has become more and more shallow since — [Client's name] work. What are you experiencing?" "[Name], it looks like some intense energy is building inside you. What do you need right now? What would be helpful to do right now?" "It looks like you are struggling to stay present. Tell me what you are thinking, feeling, experiencing?" Another one might be: "[Name], gently put your hand on the very top center of your head and look at me." Wait a few breaths and then ask: "What do you notice now?" Having someone in distress put their hand gently on top of their head center can calm them down.

For veterans and civilians in a safe group setting, be direct, look at and speak directly to another person rather than to others about them. Do this whether in person, in a group or online, as in a Zoom call. Make statements rather than ask questions, for example: instead of "Why do we have to be vulnerable in here?" State: "I do not like feeling vulnerable and having others see me that way?" Do not interpret, instead describe what you see, hear or experience and say how you feel about it. Instead of saying: "You are really angry." Instead say, "Your face is very red and you are getting louder and louder. That scares me." Here you see the focus changes from the angry person to the one who is scared. Paraphrase: restate in your own words what you heard someone say with the same emotion. This way you both get feedback.

There are many different ways to work with someone in therapy but what stays constant is being with them fully in the moment. If they are struggling with parts of themselves, such as adult with child, parent with child, or a part of self that shows up in dream as someone else, you can do a gestalt with them. Put the other part or person in a chair, or on a different pillow if you work with floor pillows. This is like what I described earlier when I was in the group and was told to put Johnny in the other chair. In doing that kind of work, you guide the process. For starters, have the veteran/client talk to whoever is in the other chair or on the other pillow. Once that is complete, have the veteran/client move to the other position by saying, "now sit on the other pillow" or "switch." From the other position, "be that part of you and respond to what was said," or "be that person and respond..." Most people are capable of intuitively going into that place and being able to accurately respond, especially if they do not think about it a lot, ask a lot of questions, and stay in their head.

You can facilitate the client talking to an actual parent of theirs and go back and forth until there is some positive change or resolution. For example: Client to parent in other chair/pillow: "Whenever I was in emotional distress as a child, you always seemed cold and disconnected from me instead of compassionate and supportive. Tell me what was going on with you?" Here the client goes to the other chair/pillow and your instructions are to: "go all the way into your parent and be her/him and respond from there, trust yourself." Another optional question: "You never seemed to show caring for me or gave nurture to me. Tell me what was going on for you or what stopped you?" (Reminder to not ask "why" questions. Consider which question you could more easily respond to: "Why did you never show me affection or nurture me?" or "You never seemed to show caring for me or gave nurture to me. Tell me what was going on for you or what stopped you?"

Using the Gestalt method with chairs or pillow, talk to a younger part of you, for example: "You seem to have a lot of fears right now. Tell me what you can about those fears." Then the therapist will say "switch" and you go to the other chair/pillow or position. From there go all the way into the fearful child and speak from there. Trust that the words and understanding will rise up inside you so you can speak it. Focus inside where your heart is, not up in your head. Intend that you will listen deeply to what is coming up.

This method can be used between any two or more people, alive or not. A veteran can do this with a deceased buddy, a deceased soldier who when last seen was suffering with horrific injuries.

If you are working with someone who is very critical and hard on themselves, they can put their critical inner parent in the other chair or pillow and have them communicate. Often when I have done this, I discover a child between 10-13 who was thrust into the job of parenting and is still doing their best in that role, but it's not at all helpful to the adult person I am working with. As the therapist, I can talk directly to this child/parent and learn what their feelings and needs are so we can come up with a way to move forward that is beneficial to them and the adult.

Because of my background, I used TA (Transactional Analysis) theory. TA theory works with ego states of the inner parent, adult, and child. Then, within the child are both different and similar structures of parent, adult and child, each with differing functions. The parent ego state has functions of structuring, nurturing, controlling, and the child has functions of natural or over adapted child, or simply OK and Not OK child, which help identify where the behavior is coming from. We can also use a simple graph based on energy. You see the balance missing in the graph. Increase S/NP and decrease controlling parent and likewise the OK and Not OK child. Shows what is going on inside.

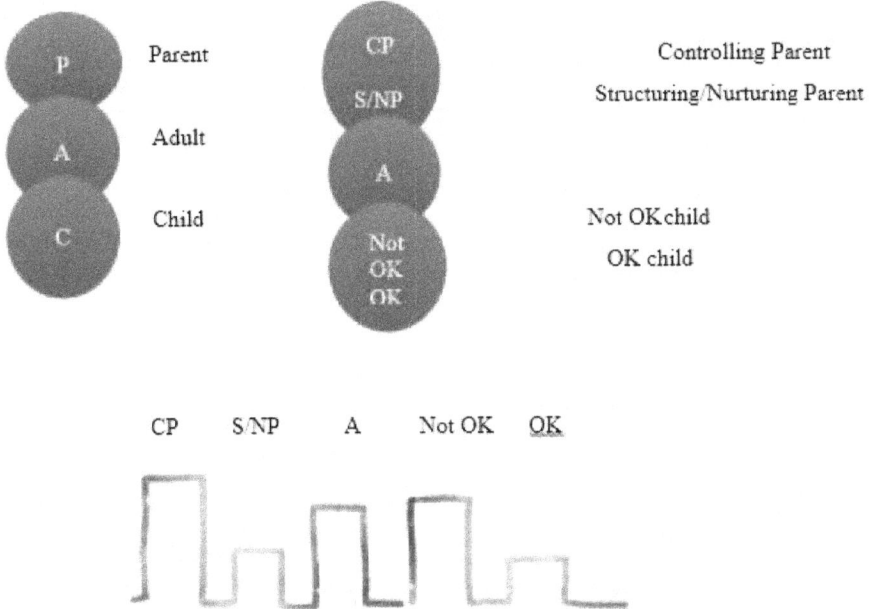

When working with people who have been traumatized, it is wise to get to a point and have them create a safe place. It can be an inside or outside place and they can determine what it looks like, where it is, what is there in the space, colors, elements, etc.

If an outside place, is it by water, trees, sand, earth, flowers, etc.? If inside, is it a large or small space, how is it decorated, what is there for your support and comfort? In all cases, this space needs to be safe from intrusion from any person or energy of any kind as in wind, rain, snow, blazing sun, locusts, predator, animal, etc. Once the person has created the safe place, have them go there, be there for a while and describe it to you.

Take notes so that, if at a time in the future when they are in a traumatic memory, you can help them go to that safe place with descriptive words. You can always say go to your safe place, but if they have not yet done so in the midst of a traumatic memory, it helps to guide them with their own description the first few times. Once they have had some practice going to and from their safe place easily while in a traumatic memory, then you can always use it when needed and so can they. Keep in mind, once you open up the memories, a trigger can bring them back to a traumatic situation in memory and it is helpful if they know how to go to their safe place on their own.

Time now to introduce you to EFT. Emotional Freedom Technique was developed by Gary Craig, who is a Stanford engineering graduate and an ordained minister. He studied with Dr. Roger Callahan who taught Thought Field Therapy but had too many complicated formulas for Gary's intentions.

Here is a description in my own words from my training of what EFT is. The brain and body do not know the difference between past and present. All the wartime/trauma memories, including sense stimuli, live in the cells of the body. Anything can trigger the release of the memories with full intensity. Those triggers are unpredictable and catch us or the veteran off guard. Once triggered, we/they can relive the trauma as though it is currently happening. They are no longer in current physical reality. Trauma leads to the need to control the environment, yet when there are many unpredictable triggers, it adds to the stress and distress the client or the veteran experiences.

When the limbic system is constantly overwhelmed, the veteran does not have access to their ability to think, problem-solve and act rationally. EFT neutralizes the chemical and physiological reactions in the body to traumatic memories and pain. Trauma and anxiety disrupt the flow of energy through the body and EFT restores the balance. EFT can also reprogram subconscious beliefs.

EFT can rewire the disturbing memories that recur from trauma and break the connection between the memories and body reactions. Symptoms are caused by a disruption in the energy system and EFT restores balance. EFT can reduce symptoms of anxiety, depression, panic, insomnia, headaches, and feeling out of control. It creates a feeling of calm and restores more normal functioning.

My suggestion is to watch the video at the following site and see the power of EFT and learn the techniques. I will put my simple protocol in the appendix and give you a link here for the newer Gold Standard techniques. https://www.dailymotion.com/video/x36qfeh https://www.practical-personal-development-advice.com/eft-for-war-veterans.html

EFT has been used to effectively treat war veterans and active military with PTSD. In a 2013 Trusted Source study, researchers studied the impact of EFT on veterans with PTSD against those receiving standard care. Within a month, participants receiving EFT coaching sessions had significantly reduced their psychological stress. In addition, more than half of the EFT test group no longer fit the criteria for PTSD. There are also some success stories from people with anxiety using EFT tapping as an alternative treatment.

A 2016 Trusted Source review compared the effectiveness of using EFT tapping over standard care options for anxiety symptoms. The study concluded there was a significant decrease in anxiety scores compared to participants receiving other care. However, further research is needed to compare EFT treatment with other cognitive therapy techniques.

EFT tapping is an alternative acupressure therapy treatment used to restore balance to your disrupted energy. It's been an authorized treatment for war veterans with PTSD and it has demonstrated some benefits as a treatment for anxiety, depression, physical pain, and insomnia. https://www.healthline.com/health/eft-tapping#research

Here is a link to the movie: Operational Emotional Freedom: The Answer: https://www.youtube.com/watch?v=hEpU9YRrGN0 The protocol/steps for EFT are in the appendix on page 250.

EMDR, Eye Movement Desensitization Reprocessing, is another method helpful to know and use with people who have a history of trauma. I have never used EMDR as therapy, but rather as a tool to use within therapy. I also use EFT when needed during the use of EMDR. If during EMDR, the recipient accesses a trauma and it is too intense for them, I use EFT to reduce the intensity and then determine whether or not to continue using EMDR during that session. Many people do not need the EFT and can go into and through the trauma without it, but it is handy to use as a tool when needed.

Here is a description of EMDR both for therapists and survivors. EMDR was designed to facilitate the accessing and processing of traumatic memories and painful life experiences and to create an adaptive resolution such that the affective distress is relieved, negative beliefs are reformulated, and physiological arousal is reduced. EMDR therapy uses a three-pronged protocol: (1) the past events that have laid the groundwork for dysfunction are processed, forging new associative links with adaptive information; (2) the current circumstances that elicit distress are targeted, and internal and external triggers are desensitized; (3) imaginal templates of future events are incorporated, to assist the client in acquiring the skills needed for adaptive functioning.

EMDR therapy shows that the mind can, in fact, heal from psychological trauma much as the body recovers from physical trauma. When you cut your hand, your body works to close the wound. If a foreign object or repeated injury irritates the wound, it festers and causes pain. Once the block is removed, healing resumes. EMDR therapy demonstrates that a similar sequence of events occurs with mental processes. The brain's information processing system naturally moves towards mental health. If the system is blocked or imbalanced by the impact of a disturbing event, the emotional wound festers and can cause intense suffering. Once the block is removed, healing resumes. Using the detailed protocols and procedures learned in EMDR training sessions, clinicians help clients activate their natural healing processes. (https://www.emdr.com/what-is-emdr/)

EMDR is extremely valuable to get as close to the actual trauma as possible to discharge all the negative energy that the trauma created. Then there is no post-traumatic stress (PTS). There are practitioners deployed to major disasters in the world who use EMDR to help people in the midst of the event so as to process it as completely as possible and reduce symptoms of PTS afterwards.

In the early 1990s, I studied Past Life Therapy and was part of a training program for several years with the Association for Past Life Research and Therapy. In my private practice I did past life therapy for those who asked for it or needed it. I may write about that in a future book, but for now I will say that it is possible to release and heal trauma from other lifetimes. I have done that for myself during the training program and for others in my work. That said, during EMDR with me, many people have been drawn into past life trauma and EMDR was just as effective, regardless of which lifetime. I think of trauma like sagebrush, a bundle of inter-connected tiny branches difficult to unravel. The EMDR process makes it easier to unravel the trauma and all that is connected to it, regardless of whether it is from your current lifetime or one that your soul lived before, that you may or may not be aware of.

I am not talking about past life regression. In regression work, the soul goes back to any particular lifetime to learn from it. In past life therapy, we specifically go back to any lifetime where there was trauma. Often, we are going back on a core issue such as abandonment. We would then look for lifetimes where the personality was abandoned and it was traumatic. We would go into each lifetime where that occurred and heal each one, which would ultimately heal that core issue of abandonment. That can be done with any core issue, including rejection, depression, scarcity etc. I once worked with a man in therapy for a few years who was doing well but had what I referred to as an overlay of depression. Going back with him lead all the way back to biblical times. It turns out he had many horrifically painful lives where he was imprisoned in some way. Once we were able to heal the very old lifetimes where he was in despair for years, and move forward to any others where he was depressed, all of his depressive symptoms were gone in his present day.

Past Life Therapy is actual therapy with the soul of the person coming in for help. Healing at the soul level can involve more than one person. I remember a woman who came to me specifically for past life therapy. We were doing therapy twice a month on her past lives and at one point she came in and asked if we could do that kind of work on someone in her life now. She described a co-worker who seemed to exude hatred toward her and she wanted to find out more about that. I took her back to a lifetime she had with that co-worker. It turned out that my client was a male in the previous life we were looking at, and the co-worker was a female. In that past lifetime, my client had her co-worker sold into slavery. The two souls had not been near each other since, but clearly the co-worker had some memory of it at the soul level, while my client did not. The therapy we did involved bringing the two souls together at a high vibrational level so my client's soul could make amends and restore balance. The proof of the effect came in phone calls I received following the therapy with them. My client called, ecstatic over the change in the co-worker the very next day. There was no longer hatred energy associated with their interactions at work. The next day, the co-worker brought a card to my client and the day afterwards gave her flowers. This kind of powerful effect occurs when we work at the soul level and the healing is instantaneous.

Another effective method useful to heal trauma is psychodrama. Psychodrama cannot be done in one-to-one therapy; it requires a group. In psychodrama you need what are called auxiliaries to take different roles. The client is asked to choose a director which could be the therapist or co-therapist. The director and client then talk together out loud so everyone can hear and see as the client describes the scene they wish to focus on. In the discussion they determine where it takes place, the set up and how that will work in the therapy space. They also determine the roles needed and the client will ask other group members if they will play a particular role the client decides suits them. Once that is complete, the client will play each role in turn to show the body postures and speak the words with the emotion needed. That way, the auxiliary role player is given a picture to copy with words and emphasis. Then they try out the role and the client gives feedback or makes changes as needed. When all the roles are set, the director sets the scene and directs the timing of which role speaks, when, and guides the client into the state they need to be in for this to unfold.

In one psychodrama, the client described the scene to the director, the family is at the dinner table. The father is loud and controlling and requires silence at the table. The children are age four and eight. The mother does not like the fact that the children cannot share their experiences at the table and does her best to eat in silence while making eye contact with the children. At one point the four-year-old boy blurts out something, stimulated by his fear. The father turns red in the face, puffs up and abruptly stands up and moves to where his son is sitting and hits him on the head while yelling. The boy turns white, stops breathing and after a pause starts to cry.

Before beginning the psychodrama to be played out in the group, the therapist regressed him to age four. The client was that boy and now he is that boy again. Once again, he is at the table with his family and when he speaks up, the father becomes red in the face, puffs up in anger and comes toward him with his arm raised. The man/boy is back there in an instant, but the father does not actually hit him now, even though he did in the actual experience. As the psychodrama plays out, the energy and emotion build and the action stops as the father raises his hand but before he hits the boy. The client does not need that part of the past to reconnect to the trauma. He stops breathing and is terrified. Then the therapist came in and held him, acting as his mother, or his mother in the scene can do the same, he tried to breathe and then cried. The important thing is that he felt safe, protected, supported and nurtured. When his emotions settled down and he talked, he used his words to describe what he was feeling and needing.

Other potential interventions that can take place are: the mother can be empowered further and insist that the family move away from the table and process what took place, each sharing their feelings and needs. At that point, they can problem solve and create a new structure for dinner at the table so family members can talk while at dinner. If the father needs the talking to be before or after eating, they can experiment with trying that out for a few days and then regroup and assess. Another option is the therapist can intervene and support the family moving away from the table and process until a new plan is developed. Yet another option is for the therapist to coach the mother so the family can move away from the table and process.

Psychodrama is a very action oriented, useful method to work with trauma resolution and there are many useful options. A client can have someone in the group agree to play the role of the client as a child. The client can then either observe with support from the therapist, or the client can become the nurturing structuring parent for the child. When the client is able to be their own nurturing/structuring parent it is a powerful moment they can build on until they are able to do that in their daily life. Clients are taught to be in touch with their inner child and that child's feelings and needs on a regular basis. When they also learn to be a structuring/nurturing parent with that child, they are able to listen and support their own inner child when the child's needs and feelings become activated. Often with veterans and others who were traumatized, they have either a traumatized inner child as well or their inner child has some strong needs and feelings that need to be acknowledged and dealt with.

It is essential to get to as many layers as possible of trauma and unexpressed feelings and needs. It is through the relationship between the client and therapist and the developed trust between them, all that can take place. You, as therapist, do not have to know all that is there, but you do have to be willing to call it up and stay with the client through all that comes with it. Clients will show or tell you what they need and if you are tuned in and listening, open and creative, you can come up with ways to fill that need. Much of the therapy that I did, came from clients who had gone through the process themselves and created a way to get their needs met that were appropriate and therapeutic.

Guided imagery is another tool that is very useful in this kind of therapy. I created one for the inner child who had intense needs and feelings, needed nurturing and structure so that the adult client could do what they needed. This one is for the journey to the crystal palace. I do this one directly with the inner child that is troubled or the adult who takes that child.

"Close your eyes and imagine that you are in a beautiful meadow, the sun is shining and you are drawn to a big oak tree. As you walk to the oak tree you see a pathway beside it and walk on it. Soon you begin to notice crystals along the edges of the path. The crystals are small but visible to you. As you walk, they seem to get bigger. The crystals are clear, different pastel colors, and all point up. You keep walking on the path and when the crystals are very large, you look ahead and start to see something gleaming brightly further up the path. When you finally arrive, you see a wide set of glistening crystalline steps. As you begin to climb up the steps, you see a plateau area up ahead and walk across it, only to come to yet another set of wide crystalline steps which you climb easily. As you get to the top, you see the smiling faces of wispy spiritual looking beings who greet you by name and welcome you to the crystal palace. One of them takes you by the hand and tells you they are taking you on a tour so you can see what is there and decide where you wish to go first. The first stop on the tour is where the food is. It is a large room with other children, some looking like you and some eating. There are small windows along the walls and in each window is something yummy to eat and even a description of it. There are so many windows it could take a long time to see it all. So far, you like everything you see and know you can't eat all of it but it is nice to know they have so many wonderful foods to choose that you can enjoy anytime you visit. You take your time and keep looking while making a mental note of the ones you like the most and where they are. You notice they all have numbers with them so you can remember the numbers of your favorites. Your tour guide gives you an electronic tablet that allows you to write freestyle or with keys. You start making a list of the foods you like the most. When you have looked at everything—you notice another wall with more food and go over there. Finally, you choose two things, one to eat and one to drink. Your tour guide asks if you would like to visit with them while you eat or visit with some of the other kids? For the moment you choose to learn more about the tour guide. When you have finished your food and drink, the tour guide points out someone who looks like an elf and will come and clear your table so you can continue your tour.

Next, you are taken to a nurture room. It is decorated with satin looking pastel-colored drapes and cozy pillows, rocking chairs and more of those wispy guides who look like your tour guide. The guides in the nurture room are sitting on pillows holding young children or in rocking chairs doing the same. There is soft music playing in the background and you see some babies in cribs sleeping. Next, you go to the music room. There you see all kinds of instruments from many different time periods all the way back and up to modern day. Each instrument comes with instructions on how it was made and from what time period and there is a recording of what it sounds like. You look around and see other children of all ages with guides who are teaching them to play various instruments. There are also soundproof side rooms where that is also going on. Next, you go to the library and it too is full of books from all the way back to when books were first printed. You also see coloring books, comic books and talking books. Wow!

This is an awesome place to visit and still there is more. You go to the control room and it looks like you are on a space ship and you can look out and see space, other planets, stars, and so much more. Your guide tells you that when you wish, you can come to the control room and learn how everything works and have a chance to fly the ship. You think to yourself that this place is heavenly and you can't wait to spend more time here. There is one more place to see for now. It is a room that is like a time machine and in it you can sit on a magic carpet and fly to anywhere you wish to go and any time period. You can do that by yourself or take a guide with you. Your guide says that for now, the tour is over and she/he will take you back to where you started. You are full of joy at all you saw and full of anticipation for what you have not yet seen or experienced there in the crystal palace. You say goodbye and look again at all the guides, wave goodbye and start down the crystal stairs. When you get to the bottom, you see the pathway and take it all the way back to the oak tree and the meadow."

Once the child has this first experience with the crystal palace, they are open to visiting whenever the adult needs them to be taken care of. The adult client can either take them there and pick them up later or the child can go on their own. This allows the child and the adult to get their needs met and neither has to suffer. If an adult has an interview or test of some sort and the child is very anxious, the adult can take the child to the crystal palace and pick them up later. Here is a link to this guided imagery I made for you. (You may have to download this to listen) https://drive.google.com/file/d/134rw_CT3AMCASbhe58qIfrSA6aSPXABj/view?usp=sharing.

Another guided imagery that I have used is to the friendly forest. "Close your eyes and imagine that you are six-years-old, in a log cabin by yourself. You look out the window in front and see beautiful tall green trees and sunshine. Then you look in the back and see a half door. The bottom is wood and the top is open but has another half with windows. You go out the door and find yourself on an earthen pathway. You begin to walk up the earthen pathway and feel the sun shining brightly on your head and shoulders. You also see some trees along the path (use seasonal visuals as in fall or spring) with blossoms on them and you hear birds singing. You are feeling happy and adventurous and see a grassy hill beside the path and go off to the right onto that grassy hill. As you climb, you feel the strength of your legs and feel the warmth of the sun and hear the songs of the birds. You keep climbing and soon you see a wooden sign stuck in the grass. You look at the sign and try to make out what is says but the letters are curly and you are not sure. As you continue to climb, you see a lot of trees up ahead and you remember hearing once about a place called the *Friendly Forest* and think about that sign and start to think this might be it. You climb the rest of the way to the top of the hill and see all the trees but as you get closer, you see that each tree has a face on its trunk and they are all smiling and waving their branches. Then you hear them singing your name… (in whispery voice say their name). You walk toward the trees and they bend and open up a pathway through the friendly forest for you. First you stop to admire the trees. There are trees with brown bark, some with reddish brown bark, some with white bark, some with gray bark and you notice that there are baby trees, great big giant trees and many in between. You go and touch some of them on their trunks and dance around between the trees. Then you go back to the path and walk further into the friendly forest.

Pretty soon you come to a clearing. In the clearing, the sun is shining brightly and standing there beside a large, rounded rock is someone who has known you for all of time. The one standing there looks right at you with a full-face smile and radiates joy and love. You run over to where they are and feel yourself being lifted up and held ever so gently yet firmly in the arms of love. Feel that fill you up. Hear that one whisper in your ear, 'I am so glad you are here. I have been waiting for you for a long time. Now that you are here, I hope you will come back as often as you like or need to. I will always be here for you.' And then the one holding you lets you down. You feel your feet touch the ground and look up at them and get a good look. You walk around them and look at their hair, face, clothing and feet. Then you go to the rock and put your palms on it. What do you notice when you put your palms on the rock? After that, you look around the clearing and notice that surrounding you in a circle are all the little creatures from the forest and they are smiling and waving their tails at you. You are full of joy and really like this place.

You go back to where the one is standing and once again you are lifted up and held gently yet firmly in the arms of love. The one holding you tells you it is time to go but now that you know the way, you can come back anytime you need or want to. With that, you are set back down on your feet and you turn and go back on the path through the friendly forest past all the trees and back out onto the grassy hill. When you get to the grassy hill you lay down on the grass and roll your body all the way down to the bottom; you get up joyfully, then you walk toward the right and pass the tree with the birds. Finally, you go back into the log cabin where you started and grow back up to be your adult self of today." Here is a link to this one that I made for you. (you may have to download it. https://drive.google.com/file/d/1fM1QgR8n-sSFza3okpQVi4FbLbZWC3Nz/view?usp=sharing

Two more techniques that are very healing for veterans are letters to the family from the war zone or from deployment and a welcome home ceremony. For the letters, the veteran is asked to remember back to their deployments or wartime experiences. Did they write home during that time and if so, what did they share? If they did not or did not fully, then ask them to go through their experiences and feelings and write them to this group family. They can do as many as they wish and this can be done over months of time if need be. When they do bring it in, ask the group members for a volunteer to read it aloud to the family group. All gather around and read/listen to the letter while the veteran observes. This gives the family an opportunity to hear and take in the feelings and experiences of their loved one while the veteran sees, hears and feels that and whatever is coming up inside them. This can be repeated for each letter. It also gives the family an opportunity to ask questions of the veteran.

The welcome home ceremony is important, especially for Vietnam Veterans and helps them reconnect to being home, out of the wartime situation, and accepted for having been through an ordeal that they can then share parts of. The ceremony marks a return to the family and home, creating a supportive atmosphere for the veteran to let go of what could get in the way of making a healthy transition back to civilian life or home life between deployments. Anything that you include in the ceremony as a true authentic welcome home with family and friends will be powerful and healing.

# Chapter 11
# SUPPORT AND ADJUNCTS TO THERAPY

When you are traumatized to the degree that you no longer feel like yourself and it seems like your experience of being in charge of you is gone, then you need resources to help you reclaim the authentic, alive, emotional you and your power. Some form of therapy is necessary and there are many adjuncts to therapy that will also help you deal with the trauma, the feelings, and body sensations that accompany it.

We will explore a number of those options in this chapter and you can choose which may serve you and your needs at any given time. Some may help you calm your mind and focus, some may help you uncover your stories and express them. Some may help you calm down your body, some may help you relate to others in healthier ways, and many will help you stay centered and grounded in response to images, sensations, thoughts, sounds, and smells from your trauma. Many will also help you stay present in the moment and in your feelings.

As we have already discussed, the emotional brain communicates through physical sensations and reactions — heart pounding, fast shallow breathing, stressed/strident voice, nausea or twisting in the stomach. Instead of being trapped or overwhelmed by those, you can learn to stay present, in the moment, aware of what is occurring and have choices for how to deal with them.

Van Der Kolk describes being pushed into a state of hyper or hypo arousal and becoming reactive and disorganized, flying into a rage, going into panic, or becoming numb and shutting down. "Recovery from trauma involves the restoration of executive functioning and with it, self-confidence and the capacity for playfulness and creativity." (*The Body Keeps the Score*, page 207) To do that you will need to calm the emotional brain and activate the pre-frontal cortex so you can be fully aware of what is going on inside you and *be* with it, without any reactions or judgements. Allow yourself to feel, sense, know what is happening without running from it in anyway. This is where mindfulness, movement, rhythm, marital arts, yoga, music, arts, drumming and theater come in to save the day. We will look at each one of these and have a basic understanding of each of them and how they can help you in your recovery from trauma.

## 1. MINDFULNESS

The foundation of mindfulness is awareness and acceptance. You learn how to be aware of yourself, your thoughts, feelings, sensations, and processes. You learn to track what is going on inside you, minute by minute through observation, without judgement or measurement of any kind. You are in the here and now, which is key to healing, and you are aware of all of your own thoughts, feelings, sensations, and focus, while accepting all of it, no matter what it is. Mindfulness becomes a way of life, of showing up completely in the moment and relating to yourself, others, and situations calmly and purposefully no matter what obstacles, stressors, and challenges show up. What mindfulness does is allow people to remain focused and present rather than avoiding problems. By focusing on the present moment without judging it, you can gain clarity and freedom to decide how to respond to any situation. You make the choice to focus on the present moment fully rather than be trapped in your thoughts and emotions of the past or future. You live life as it is, rather than with any judgements or expectations. It is actually easier than holding any judgements. Holding judgments takes energy and focus away from your own life.

If you find that you have many automatic reactions to people, words, facial expressions, or situations, then mindfulness will help you avoid falling victim to these automatic reactions. Using deep breathing and your senses of sight, sound, touch, and smell, you learn to stay focused in the moment, so your mind decreases activity in your sympathetic nervous system (the one responsible for the fight-or-flight stress reaction) and activates or increases energy in your parasympathetic nervous system (the one responsible for rest and calm).

When you're stuck in your mind with your thoughts and feelings going round and round, you can't see clearly what you need to do to solve the immediate problem. When you're lost in your thoughts and emotions, you also miss out on the pleasures and joys of each moment, because you're not completely aware of them. You could be in a conversation with someone and not be present so that later, that person reminds you of what you said and you will not remember because you actually were not present. Mindfulness supports you to increase a calm, neutral awareness of your thoughts, emotions, physical sensations, and behaviors.

Here are some mindfulness exercises:

**Body scan mindfulness.** Lie on your back with your legs extended and arms at your sides, palms facing up. Focus your attention slowly and deliberately on each part of your body, in order, from toe to head or head to toe. Be aware of any sensations, emotions or thoughts associated with each part of your body. Simply notice without judgement or measurement of any kind.

**Sitting meditation.** Sit comfortably with your back straight, feet flat on the floor and hands in your lap. Breathing through your nose, focus on your breath moving in and out of your body. If physical sensations, thoughts or sounds interrupt your meditation, note the experience and then return your focus to your breath.

**Walking meditation.** Find a quiet place ten to twenty feet in length, and begin to walk slowly. Focus on the experience of walking, being aware of the sensations of standing and the subtle movements that keep your balance. When you reach the end of your path, turn and continue walking, maintaining awareness of your sensations. You may be able to find some labyrinths which tend to be circular, in your local area around churches or spiritual centers.

**Mindfulness Exercises**
https://www.veteranshealthlibrary.va.gov/HealthyLiving/Stress/Mindfulness/142,85190_VA

https://www.militaryonesource.mil/resources/mobile-apps/de-stress-and-relax-with-chill-drills-by-military-onesource/

https://www.themindfulword.org/mindfulness-for-veterans/

These easy mindfulness exercises are simple enough for anyone to try, and yet they are an extraordinarily powerful method for developing self-awareness.

Mindfulness is awareness of the present moment. It's living here and now. Through mindfulness, you are freed from becoming entangled in thoughts of your past, and you are freed from worrying about the future. In the here and now, everything just is...and there is great peace in that. But, how to stay in touch with this moment, especially when your mind keeps running away from you like it so often does? If mindfulness is a new idea to you, then it might seem a little daunting to try and keep your attention fixed in the present moment, but I trust you can do it if you choose.

These mindfulness techniques are an important part of learning how to practice mindfulness.

*Exercise 1: One Minute of Mindfulness*
This is an easy mindfulness exercise, and one that you can do anytime throughout the day. Take a moment right now to try this. Check your watch and note the time. For the next sixty, seconds your task is to focus all your attention on your breathing. It's just for one minute, but it can seem like an eternity. Leave your eyes open and breathe normally. Be

ready to catch your mind from wandering off (because it will) and return your attention to your breath whenever it does so.

This mindfulness exercise is far more powerful than most people give it credit for. It takes some people many years of practice before they are able to complete a single minute of alert, clear attention.

Keep in mind that this mindfulness exercise is not a contest or a personal challenge. You can't fail at this exercise you can only experience it. Use this exercise many times throughout the day to restore your mind to the present moment and to restore your mind to clarity and peace. Over time, you can gradually extend the duration of this exercise into longer and longer periods. This exercise is actually the foundation of a correct mindfulness meditation technique.

You can also use a mindfulness bell to focus your attention on, instead of your breathing. If you have struggled with mantra meditations or breathing meditation techniques in the past, then a mindfulness bell recording can really help you to focus your attention in the present moment and achieve a state of mental stillness. Here is a description of an app that plays a mindfulness bell. Enjoy on your iPhone, iPad, and iPod. It rings a beautiful Tibetan Singing Bowl at a specified interval - or random intervals - throughout the day. The sound of these beautiful bells can help bring you back to your true center - and back into the present moment. https://www.youtube.com/watch?v=4ubvtvQFTlo

### *Exercise 2: Conscious Observation*

Pick up an object that you have lying around. Any mundane everyday object will do, a coffee cup or a pen for example. Hold it in your hands and allow your attention to be fully absorbed by the object. Observe it. Don't assess it or think about it, or study it intellectually. Just observe it for what it is.

You'll feel a sense of heightened "nowness" during this exercise. Conscious observation can really give you a feeling of "being awake." Notice how your mind quickly releases thoughts of past or future, and how different it feels to be in the moment. Conscious observation is a form of meditation. It's subtle, but powerful. By practicing mindfulness in this way, you'll really start to sense what mindfulness is all about.

In the book, *Mindfulness, Bliss and Beyond*, Ajahn Brahm describes his own personal experience of conscious observation:

"The mind is like a megawatt searchlight, enabling you to see so much deeper into what you are gazing at. Ordinary concrete becomes a masterpiece. A blade of grass literally shimmers with the most delightful and brilliant shades of fluorescent green...the pretty becomes profound and the humdrum becomes heavenly under the sparkling energy of power mindfulness."

You can also practice conscious observation with your ears rather than your eyes. Many people find that mindful listening is a more powerful mindfulness technique than visual observation.

### Exercise 3: The Ten Second Count

This is more of an exercise in practicing concentration than it is in mindfulness, and it is a simple variation on Exercise 1. In this exercise, rather than focusing on your breath, you simply close your eyes and focus your attention on slowly counting to ten. If your concentration wanders off, start back at number one! For most people, it goes something like this...

"One...two...three...do I have to buy milk today or did John say he'd do it? Oh, whoops, I'm thinking."

"One...two...three...four...this isn't so hard after all... Oh no....that's a thought! Start again."

"One...two...three... now I've got it. I'm really concentrating now..."

This website has some good information as well and states that meditation is one of the best mindfulness techniques. https://www.powerofpositivity.com/mindfulness-techniques-most-people-forget/

## 2. MEDITATION

Meditation is a mind and body practice that has a long history of use for increasing calmness and relaxation, quieting the mind, coping with illness and distress, and enhancing overall health and well-being. Mind and body practices focus on the connections between the brain, mind, body, and behavior.

There are many types of meditation, and most have four elements in common: a quiet location with as few distractions as possible; a specific, comfortable posture (sitting, lying down, walking, or in other positions); a focus of attention (a specially chosen word or set of words, an object, or the sensations of the breath); and an open attitude (letting distractions come and go naturally without judging them).

The Mayo Clinic says: Meditation can give you a sense of calm, peace and balance that can benefit both your emotional well-being and your overall health. And these benefits don't end when your meditation session ends. Meditation can help carry you more calmly through your day and may help you manage symptoms of certain medical conditions.

**Meditation and Emotional Well-being**
When you meditate, you may clear away the information overload that builds up every day and contributes to your stress.

The emotional benefits of meditation can include:

- Gaining a new perspective on stressful situations
- Building skills to manage your stress
- Increasing self-awareness
- Focusing on the present
- Reducing negative emotions
- Increasing imagination and creativity
- Increasing patience and tolerance

Meditation is an umbrella term for the many ways to a relaxed state of being. There are many types of meditation and relaxation techniques that have meditation components. All share the same goal of achieving inner peace.

Ways to meditate can include:

**Guided meditation.** Sometimes called guided imagery or visualization, with this method of meditation you form mental images of places or situations you find relaxing. You try to use as many senses as possible, such as smells, sights, sounds and textures. Here is link to a guided meditation you can use:
https://www.youtube.com/watch?v=y3TrGysWETw&feature=youtu.be

**Mantra meditation.** In this type of meditation, you silently repeat a calming word, thought or phrase to prevent distracting thoughts. Examples: Love, Peace, Light, Calm, Soothing.

**Mindfulness meditation.** This type of meditation is based on being mindful, or having an increased awareness and acceptance of living in the present moment. In mindfulness meditation, you broaden your conscious awareness. You focus on what you experience during meditation, such as the flow of your breath. You can observe your thoughts and emotions, but let them pass without judgment. Imagine them floating across your mind and going away.

**Loving kindness meditation.** With loving kindness meditation, the aim is to direct feelings of compassion towards yourself and others. It's easy to add this on to any basic mindfulness meditation. For example, instead of just focusing on your breath, try thinking about someone else in your head. Then, say this phrase aloud: "May you be happy. May you be healthy. May you be safe." You can direct these positive thoughts toward yourself, someone you love, or someone you don't particularly like at the moment. In fact, loving kindness meditation has been found to help improve self-esteem and even resolve conflicts.

**Walking meditation.** During walking meditation, you will focus on each step as you mindfully lift and place your foot on the ground. You can walk anywhere — a hallway inside, a sidewalk in the city, or out in a park. Walking meditation may be worth trying if you don't like sitting still for a traditional mindfulness meditation. It offers the same advantages of meditation — plus the health benefits of walking.

You may find this website helpful:
https://zenhabits.net/meditation-guide/

## 3. YOGA

The science of yoga is a 5,000-year-old system that leads to physical vitality, peace of mind, and a deepening experience of spiritual connection. The word yoga is derived from the Sanskrit root *yuj*, meaning "to yoke," or "to unite." The practice of yoga aims to create union between body, mind and spirit, as well as between the individual self and universal consciousness and to move out of ego driven thoughts.

Yoga has been practiced for thousands of years, and the goal of yoga is to achieve liberation from suffering through practices which bring together body, mind and breath as a means of altering energy or shifting consciousness. In India, it is the union between self and the divine.

Yoga is an art as well as a science. It is a science because it offers practical methods for controlling body and mind, thereby making deep meditation possible. And it is an art, for unless it is practiced intuitively and sensitively, it will yield only superficial results.

Yoga is not a system of beliefs. It takes into account the influence on each other of body and mind, and brings them into mutual harmony. So often, for instance, the mind cannot concentrate simply because of tension or illness in the body which prevent the energy from flowing to the brain. So often, too, the energy in the body is weakened because the will is dispirited or paralyzed by harmful emotions.

Yoga works primarily with the energy in the body, through the science of pranayama, or energy-control. Prana means also 'breath.' Yoga teaches how, through breath-control, to still the mind and attain higher states of awareness.

Many people begin practicing yoga as a way to cope with feelings of anxiety. Interestingly enough, there is quite a bit of research showing that yoga can help reduce anxiety. In one study, thirty-four women diagnosed with an anxiety disorder participated in yoga classes twice weekly for two months. At the end of the study, those who practiced yoga had significantly lower levels of anxiety than the control group (6Trusted Source).

Another study followed sixty-four women with post-traumatic stress disorder (PTSD), which is characterized by severe anxiety and fear following exposure to a traumatic event. After 10 weeks, the women who practiced yoga once weekly had fewer symptoms of PTSD. In fact, 52% of participants no longer met the criteria for PTSD at all (7Trusted Source).

It's not entirely clear exactly how yoga is able to reduce symptoms of anxiety. However, it emphasizes the importance of being present in the moment and finding a sense of peace, which could help treat anxiety.

## 4. EQUINE ASSISTED THERAPY

Horses by nature are hypervigilant until they learn they are not in danger. Those with PTSD are also hypervigilant and whatever their emotions, behavior or body responses will be mirrored back by the horse they are with. Horses are in the moment and require that we are as well if we are with them. They do not know your past and accept you as you are in any given moment. If you choose to do equine assisted therapy you will be required, by the horse, to learn what does and does not work when communicating with them. Equine therapy gives you the opportunity to try new communication methods with your horse.

Horses are well-suited for the therapy environment because of their natural instincts and communication methods. While humans can speak, explain, and rationalize thoughts, horses live in an entirely action-based social structure. This works well in therapy because in action-based exercises you *must* change your actions to change your results — horses don't question your motives; they react to the actions you take.

Their hyper-vigilance and heavy reliance on body language makes them valuable assets to those with PTSD. Horses are more aware of body language than humans and more easily recognize and react to levels of anger, anxiety, fear, or sadness that may be imperceptible to humans. This allows real-time feedback for the seeker and the therapist.

Equine Assisted Therapy for Veterans falls along a spectrum of modalities. Some programs teach horsemanship and riding, others are strictly interacting with the horses from the ground. Some include therapists, others don't. This gives veterans the opportunity to find a program that best fits their needs.

Erin Fristad told me, "Many of our clients express that it's more comfortable to be with the horses in the arena, than sitting in a room talking to a therapist. They also tell us the horses can detect their bullshit! Horses hold us all accountable." (Erin Fristad, Life Coach & Equine Specialist, Wild Cove Farm, erin@erinfristad.com and Info@wildcovefarm.com.

The following is from:
**https://www.equinetherapygroup.com/what-we-offer/ptsd/**
The client is given exercises and tasks to make the horse perform. It may be as simple as having the horse walk over a pole or as challenging as having it follow you through an obstacle course. The techniques that clients try with these challenges are varied and telling. The client typically has to try several different approaches (some of them very different from how they usually communicate) before finding one that the horse understands and is comfortable with. People tend to communicate with the horses in the same manner that they communicate within their relationships. If you can't get the horse to do something, you have the chance to experiment with your approach to get the desired result. Observing the client during these challenges and asking open-ended questions such as "do you think the horse understood what you were doing" or "what can you tell me about what

just happened" guides the client towards their goals but allows them to do it in their words with their strategies.

Hope for Heroes is an equine therapy consulting and horsemanship program specializing in veterans and active-duty military in Yelm, Washington, near Joint Base Lewis McChord. Founded in 2018, they serve 45 veterans and active-duty military every week, free of charge. Hope for Heroes has been working with the Army Warrior Transition Battalion and Air Force Medical Flight for the past ten years and will begin assisting the 1st Special Forces Group at JBLM in a similar capacity.

Hope for Heroes' Operations Director, Debbi Fisher and her husband Robert Woelk, Executive Director, also founded Rainier Therapeutic Riding in 2010, which served over 100 veterans and active-duty military weekly. "There's a need for more equine programs like ours in Washington State. We are already operating at close to our capacity of fifty-five participants weekly, and the area north of Seattle does not have any such programs," stresses Woelk.

The Hope for Heroes equine program teaches basic natural horsemanship with a focus on reading horse behavior, communication, and establishing a leadership role with a horse. They have no therapists on staff, nor any traditional therapy included in the lessons. The horses are their only therapists.

"We rely on a horse's natural ability to read and detect anxiety in humans and their ability to mirror this anxiety back to the participant. This immediate biofeedback is exactly what our participants require to help them relearn how to self-manage their anxiety disorder. This anxiety mirroring is extremely effective, and within four-six weeks of instruction, we see smiles and self-confidence where none existed before. All of our participants share that our program is the very best and only therapy that has helped them. Many share that their horse has saved their life, either from suicide or chronic depression. Just recently, a veteran shared that she no longer has any of the extreme nightmares that have plagued her every night for years, and that this has happened since she started our horse program eight weeks ago," shares Woelk.

"Our greatest wish is to inspire other horse enthusiasts to start an equine program for veterans in the Pacific Northwest," stresses Woelk. "Debbi and I would love to help and coach any such undertaking. The thought of putting suicidal veterans on a waiting list weighs heavy on my heart." For more information visit:
https://www.nwhorsesource.com/hope-for-heroes-equine-therapy-consulting-and-horsemanship-center/

**Other resources**:
https://www.heartofhorsesense.org http://unbridledcounseling.com
http://healingreins.com/our-tem/
https://www.operationwearehere.com/EquineTherapy.html
https://sunnycreekranch.com/horses-for-heroes
https://heartbeatforwarriors.org/therapeutic-programs/back-in-the-saddle/ http://www.blendedspiritsranch.org
https://trrhelp.org/warrior-camp/

The following is from: Military.com | By Stew Smith (https://mst.military.com/benefits/veterans-health-care/veteran-horse-therapy.html)

There is something special about the moment a 2,800-pound draft horse connects with you that requires you to be completely yourself. It is the moment that kicks off a true, honest and humbling relationship that makes you feel like the animal is bonding with your spirit or soul.

Those bonding moments continue as the relationship begins to pull the "real you" out again after years of either having lost it or hiding it as you mask the pain from the experiences of war and violence, a problem especially apparent among the tactical professions. Therapy horses are nonjudgmental and do not have expectations or motives toward the people with whom they connect. And horses have a keen ability to understand the attitudes and behaviors of the humans they meet.

## What Is Veteran Horse Therapy?
Also known as equine therapy, veteran horse therapy is simply an experimental treatment involving interactions between a veteran and a horse.

I was first exposed to horse therapy when I visited Boulder Crest Retreat (with locations in Virginia and Arizona), a veteran-focused, all-expenses paid program aimed at post-traumatic growth. The exposure to horses was easily the most impactful for me and many other veterans, and I was very impressed with the program. There are many programs available for veterans to experience this type of therapy.

## Benefits of Veteran Horse Therapy
According to CRC Health, horseback riding or equine therapy has been successful in helping patients show marked improvements in the following areas:

- Assertiveness
- Emotional awareness
- Empathy
- Stress tolerance
- Flexibility
- Impulse control
- Problem-solving skills
- Self-actualization
- Independence
- Self-regard
- Social responsibility
- Interpersonal relationships
- Post-traumatic stress
- Traumatic Brain Injury (TBI)

## 5. SERVICE DOGS
Service dogs are specifically and highly trained to assist military veterans in achieving better quality of life. Veterans who utilize service

dogs report lower levels of depression and anxiety, fewer hospitalizations and a reduction in medical and psychiatric costs. Service dog benefits include:

- Ease loneliness and stress
- Reduce social anxiety
- Decrease reliance on prescription drugs
- Help veterans return to work or attend college
- Strengthen personal relationships
- Provide security, protection and unconditional love

Veterans have reported that service dogs reduced their hypervigilance by alerting them of potential danger, creating boundaries, disrupting nightmares, improving sleep quality and duration. Dogs also helped veterans turn their attention away from invasive trauma-related thoughts. Other reported benefits include: improved emotional connections with others, increase in community participation, greater physical activity, and reduction in their suicidal impulses and medication use.

Veterans said that service dogs help reduce PTSD symptoms and facilitated their recovery and achieving meaningful goals. Service dogs may be a reasonable option for veterans who are reluctant to pursue or persist with traditional evidence-based treatments.

Veterans with PTSD are hyper-vigilant about their safety, and service dogs can make them feel safer by entering the home before them and turning on the lights with a foot pedal. These dogs can also help PTSD sufferers who feel overwhelmed in public places by creating a physical barrier between the handler and others, giving the handler more personal space. Many PTSD sufferers find that having a service dog to care for forces them to also take care of themselves, by getting out into the world and getting exercise with their dog.

Service dogs offer a unique, non-judgmental, ever present comfort. More importantly, they serve as an early alert system to mood swings and emotional changes, enabling the individual to engage in positive coping strategies and lessening the severity of these symptoms by offering a variety of calming behaviors. The consistency of the service dog also eases fear of the unknown, because the service dog is always available to go for help or retrieve medication if needed.

PTSD service dogs have been useful for anyone with the following symptoms: anxiety, panic, fear, irritability, depression, withdrawal, isolation, hyper-vigilance, loss of trust, nightmares, reoccurring flashbacks, phobias of crowds, phones, e-mail, stores, buildings, vehicles, unfamiliar people, insomnia, fatigue, pounding heart, migraines, difficulty concentrating, paranoia, sleepwalking, suicidal thoughts, anti-social behavior, suspicion, and poor self-esteem.

## 6. WRITING

Ron Capps founded the Veterans Writing Project in North Carolina and hung a hand-lettered sign next to his desk which read, "Either you control the memory or the memory controls you." This and the following are from Ron Capps:
(https://www.veteranswriting.org/work)

Since its inception nine years ago, the project has provided no-cost writing and songwriting workshops to veterans and their family members. So far, the program has reached 5,000 people in 22 states. "Every veteran has a story," says Capps, 61, who served in Afghanistan, Kosovo, Rwanda, Darfur and Iraq. "Most of us, though, need help in telling that story."

That is where writing programs come in. A teacher/guide works with the group members, gives assignments, helps process the writing and supports the process that each veteran goes through over the time they are in the program. There are many programs in cities and towns all over the U.S.

In another program in Asheville, North Carolina, almost every veteran when asked to participate said they "couldn't write." It turns out that they all could, and did. They used "prompts" ... short pieces, poems, or stories that open a topic to encourage thinking, writing, and a basis for dialogue. The work continued at home at their own pace.

There is no bad writing, no wrong way to do so. There is no judgment, only acceptance, encouragement and support. It requires only honesty and a willingness to find a new kind of courage.

We've held three writing groups over the past two years, all successful beyond what we could have imagined. Each veteran reported significant improvement in their symptoms or quality of life. For many it's been transformative, as it has been for those privileged to lead the work. The groups have become a brotherhood around new shared experience.
(https://www.veteranswriting.org/work)


The following is from
https://www.huffpost.com/entry/ptsd-veterans-writing_b_1078971

Telling our stories helps us heal. It releases some of the energy the experience created and helps to externalize the experience. In telling our story, it is not ours alone. Someone is sharing it with us. In enabling another to understand and have empathy, we move out of isolation toward the experience of community, a requirement for healing.

In the last twenty years, medical practice has increasingly recognized the importance of "narrative medicine." Many medicalschools now have Narrative Medicine programs.
https://www.huffpost.com/entry/ptsd-veterans-writing_b_1078971

https://www.facebook.com/warriorwriters.org This group meets first and third Fridays at a specific time depending on location. For me, Sarah, it is 9:30-11:30 a.m. We are given a prompt and we write silently for twenty or so minutes and then share what we wrote. This is a great accepting group.

On the website https://www.theredbadgeproject.com, it states, "For Wounded Warriors struggling to heal the invisible wounds of PTSD, anxiety and depression, believing in the value of their story and finding the means to communicate it to family, friends and community is a struggle of heroic proportions. Our stories inform the audacity of the imagination and the understanding of ourselves as unique individuals."

The Red Badge Project founders, Evan Bailey and veteran and actor Tom Skerritt, talk about their experiences and vision for healing trauma through the arts. The project encourages soldiers to rediscover their personal voices using the fundamentals of storytelling. Skip Nichols from Walla Wall said he "learned to put the words down on paper as I felt them, … this writing healed me or has helped heal me and I don't know if I'd be here if it wasn't for Red Badge. And I mean that sincerely. There are too many veterans coming back now that are withdrawing and they need to be able to share their experiences in words and on paper and ultimately with you so that we can prevent more wounded veterans."

Using the fundamentals of Storytelling, in concert with current military psychiatric programs, The Red Badge Project encourages soldiers to rediscover self-trust, to believe in the value of their experiences, and to realize that theirs is a story worth telling, in their own voice. Participants discover greater self-acceptance and efficacy as they find their voice, and produce stories inspired by their life experiences. They understand the creative process and utilize a variety of tools to express themselves within and beyond the classroom. Participants feel safe within and beyond the classroom through outreach to participants' families, peers and the larger community. (https://www.theredbadgeproject.com/category/student-productions/page/2/)

From
https://usvaa.org/program-the-usvaa-veterans-writing-program/

The United States Veterans Artist Alliance strives to address issues of concern to veterans and their families via artistic endeavors and platforms. These issues include the transition from military to civilian life, education, employment, the effects of wartime and military service injuries such as PTSD, TBI and Military Sexual Trauma (MST) and homelessness among veterans. They do writer's workshops periodically.

Here are some comments about one of them:

*"USVAA has been instrumental in my transition from being an Air Force Officer to becoming a working television writer. The mentors have provided nothing short of phenomenal guidance and honest feedback when it came to making my writing shine. I owe my confidence in my own writing abilities to USVAA."*

**Jalysa Conway, veteran, USAF, Staff Writer/Story Editor, Grey's Anatomy**

The following quote is from Kadyn Michaels noted below.

*"Through the mentorship of the USVAA professional volunteers, I have been able to develop my craft as a writer in an environment that is both artistically safe and professionally exacting. As an emerging writer, access to such an environment cannot be underestimated or over appreciated."*

**Kadyn Michaels, Finalist, 2018 Francis Ford Coppola Screenwriting Competition**

USVAA has worked with the Writers Guild Foundation (WGF) since the first year of their Veterans Writing Program in 2010. They are proud to collaborate on their annual Veterans Writing Weekend Retreat as part of their overall mission to assist veterans through professional development in the arts, humanities and the entertainment industry.

The WGF program is a phenomenal success and has provided USVAA with a structured and unique opportunity to conduct a series of ongoing monthly writing workshops at their theater in Culver City to further develop the writing talent of the veterans with whom they work. Here is their contact information: USVAA, Keith Jeffreys Executive Director (310) 397-4500 keith.jeffreys@usvaa.org

The mission of the Writers Guild Foundation's Veterans Writing Project is to identify emerging writers from United States military backgrounds and provide them with the tools and insights to nurture their passion for writing and successfully navigate the entertainment industry.

They do this in two phases over a yearlong program: A weekend-long retreat, and monthly follow-up workshops and special events. Each military veteran is paired with WGA members. Their writer-mentors represent some of the most beloved movies and television series of the past and present, and are committed to guiding the voices of the future. From their website: https://usvaa.org/program-the-usvaa-veterans-writing-program/

**PATH WITH ART** TRANSFORMS THE LIVES OF PEOPLE RECOVERING FROM HOMELESSNESS, ADDICTION, AND OTHER TRAUMA BY HARNESSING THE POWER OF CREATIVE ENGAGEMENT AS A BRIDGE TO COMMUNITY AND A PATH TO STABILITY.

This program is in the Seattle area as well as online, and has a veteran cohort, programs specifically for veterans. Their programming involves different forms of writing, different art forms and music. All classes are free and open to all with low income. Those leading the programs and those assisting are helpful to anyone attending and support them having a successful experience. Each quarter there are different classes, and you can sign up for whichever program calls to you. They have classes at The Art Home in Seattle and many are also on Zoom. Path With Art has many varied programs for veterans including writing, different art forms, music, and more all the time. See website and look under programs then veterans: https://www.pathwithart.org

Path with Art (PWA) works in concert with the Seattle Opera. In 2019, the Veterans Chorus with male and female veterans from Vietnam to post 911, were part of the Opera, The Falling and Rising at Tagney Jones Hall, Seattle Opera. In November 2023, the veterans chorus sang along with the U.S. Soldier's Chorus at Tagney Jones Hall, Seattle Opera. In December 2023, Path With Art, held a Showcase so that participant artists could show what they accomplished in their classes that quarter. I was in a songwriting class and wrote my first song which I was able to sing at the showcase. I also participated in the veteran's chorus and the band. Because of support from the Seattle Opera, I was given a free music therapy session. In that session I told the therapist that I missed drumming, as I had been an African drummer as part of an ensemble for over ten years. I could not do it anymore because of pain in my fingers and wrist. She put several large stand- up drums in front of me and handed me some mallets. I had a great time playing those drums and realized I could drum with sticks. I found some fatter drum sticks with cotton balls on the ends and I can play a Dun Dun and Sang Ban with them in the PWA Band and at the music jams.

## 7. MUSIC, ART, THEATER

Warrior Songs has spent most of the past decade using songwriting and other artistic endeavors to assist veterans with PTSD help channel the flood of emotions they experience after returning from battle. Warrior Songs is a non-profit organization committed to facilitating veterans' healing through music and the creative arts.

The organization was started by Jason Moon, an Iraq War veteran who returned to Wisconsin in 2004 from a tour of duty and found it difficult to adjust to civilian life while suffering from post-traumatic stress disorder. "I had a hard time," Moon told Fox News. "I didn't know it at the time, but I had PTSD. For four years, I just went downhill." Life became increasingly dire. In 2008 he attempted suicide. That was the moment that led him to seek help.

He went for observation at his local VA hospital and when he was released, he looked for ways to deal with the pain he carried. "I started writing songs," he said. "They were really supposed to be cathartic for me. It was really the best way to get all that stuff off my chest."

In 2011, he compiled the songs he wrote into an album titled "Trying to Find My Home." After posting the music online, he received e-mails from other vets and their family members telling him how his music helped them with their own process.

Moon decided to go on the road and perform for others in the veteran community. During this time, he became inspired to start Warrior Songs. "Once I realized my music was helping other people, I felt it was worth sticking with and that I had to help others."

Processing those experiences through music or other artistic mediums helps to bridge the gap between vets and their loved ones and also helps them reclaim hope. Through artistic retreats where they write songs, create visual art, and most importantly, experience camaraderie with other vets — perhaps the only other people who understand what they went through. Ray, a Vietnam Veteran said: "It's been over forty years since my return from the conflict in Vietnam, for the first time I've felt acceptance among my peers. I feel that my isolation, failed relationships and sketchy career have been vindicated in the truth telling of our stories, my experiences have been validated. Now I am free to speak my truth because of you all, able to accept my place as 'elder,' no longer a pariah. Through art, through poetry, song and writing, Warrior Songs has made it possible to speak the unspeakable."

A younger veteran said: "You come back to civilian life and people just don't care," he said. "It makes things difficult and you just want to give up." In 2013, he attended a Warrior Songs retreat where he wrote his own songs about the pain he went through and gained solace in the camaraderie with other vets. "It wasn't until I went to the retreat that I was able to open up. I was unable to do that for a long time. It gave me the opportunity to express where I've been and help me through it." https://www.warriorsongs.org/creative-arts-healing-retreats

## Art Therapy

One of the most exciting things taking place in the field of art therapy is in the area of treating our veterans with PTSD, TBI, and other psychological health conditions. Over and over again, we hear amazing stories about how the art therapist working with vets has changed their lives forever. National Endowment of the Arts (NEA) in partnership with the U.S. Department of Defense and Veterans Affairs, plus state and local arts agencies places creative arts therapies at the core of patient-centered care at eleven military medical facilities across the country, as well as a telehealth program to reach patients in rural and remote areas, and increase access to therapeutic arts activities for military personnel and their families in local communities.

https://www.arts.gov/initiatives/creative-forces

Chris Stowe, a veteran interviewed by Karen Pence, Second Lady, said: "I can say without reservation that art therapy saved my mental health, my marriage, and ultimately my life. I was on the verge of giving up on ever getting better until I found art therapy. I continue to use art therapy to this day."

Art therapy uses creative mediums like drawing, painting, coloring, and sculpture. For PTSD recovery, art helps process traumatic events in a new away. Art provides an outlet when words fail. With a trained art therapist, every step of the therapy process involves art. Erica Curtis, a licensed marriage and family therapist, said, "I help clients identify coping strategies and internal strengths to begin the journey of healing; they may create collages of images representing internal strengths," she explains.

Adds Curtis: "When you bring art or creativity into a session, on a very, very basic level, it taps into other parts of a person's experience. It accesses information … or emotions that maybe can't be accessed through talking alone." She also says: "Just like art can bridge feelings and words, it can also be a bridge back into feeling grounded and safe in one's body."

Because people who were traumatized often do not feel safe in their bodies, art therapy is a way to help them reconnect to their body and feelings while creating safety. Look for an art therapist to work with that is knowledgeable in the integration of trauma-based approaches and theories. A trauma informed therapist.

Clients examine feelings and thoughts about trauma by making a mask or drawing a feeling and discussing it. Art can build grounding and coping skills by photographing pleasant objects. It can help tell the story of trauma by creating a graphic timeline. Through methods like these, integrating art into therapy addresses a person's whole experience. This is critical with PTSD.

One form of art therapy/expression is Touch Drawing. Many retreats for veterans include art and musical forms of expression. Explore online for veteran retreat options that appeal to you. There are many for men and some for women veterans. I am personally connected to The Highground in Wisconsin https://www.thehighground.us and have been facilitating women veteran retreats there for a couple of years. In a recent retreat in June of 2022, a woman veteran let herself go deep into her trauma and released a lot of it through her drawings and drumming. She is much more empowered now and feeling more positive about herself and her life.

Using your hands on tissue paper to create images can be very healing. For those who have been traumatized, outlets such as touch drawing, can provide release and restoration. Words are not necessary and for these people, not always readily available. Instead, the freedom to express what is inside and in your bodies, is a wonderful life changing outlet. Traumatized individuals who do not feel safe in their bodies find touch drawing a healing release and relief. Through touch drawing they can reconnect to their bodies and feelings in ways they cannot through talking.

During touch drawing, someone who was traumatized can simply tune into their body and the feelings inside them, and with support, put it all out on the paper. The thoughts and feelings maybe jumbled up inside and have no outlet until they find their hands dancing across the paper and creating images. They are not producing art— they are healing. They learn the simple basics of preparing their board, covering the paint with tissue paper and then easing into release. Touch drawing is an easy way for people to express what they fear and what is hiding inside them. Through their own hands and tuning into their bodies and feelings they can learn to heal the trauma that keeps them stuck and in pain.

Touch Drawing allows for someone's body and brain to express terror, confusion, rage, and grief in order to move into their power once again. They can also begin to create new strategies or coping skills through the images they consciously or unconsciously put on their papers. My favorite part of touch drawing is when we get into a circle after the drawings have been completed, viewed in private by the artist, and then later shared with others in the circle.

In the circle each of us is able to look at the images that came out—without judgement. I am always amazed at what shows up that was not intended. So many times, someone is simply releasing feelings but angels show up on the page, or a beloved pet, or an unknown face. When people give themselves over to the process and trust, amazing images show up and offer hope and healing. Here is the link for the center for Touch Drawing.

https://deborahkoff-chapin.com/deborah/

"Art expression is a powerful way to safely contain and create separation from the terrifying experience of trauma," writes board-certified art therapist, Gretchen Miller, for the National Institute for Trauma and Loss in Children. "Art safely gives voice to and makes a survivor's experience of emotions, thoughts, and memories visible when words are insufficient."

Using art therapy to treat PTSD addresses the whole experience of trauma: mind, body, and emotion. By working through PTSD with art, what was a terrifying experience that caused lots of symptoms can become a neutralized story from the past.

https://www.healthline.com/health/art-therapy-for-ptsd

Art can be a wonderful tool and outlet for those working through the trauma at the core of PTSD. Art therapists are trained to not only encourage artistic expression in people who might otherwise be reticent, but they are also trained in recognizing patterns of human behavior exemplified in the artwork. Art may also be used as a source of personal relief when dealing with PTSD. While it is certainly a helpful therapy modality, art does not have to be created under the eye of a certified art therapist to aid in the healing process. Simply getting the jumble of thoughts and feelings within onto paper or canvas can be immensely helpful and cathartic. Art does not have to follow any linear progression. It is not graded or evaluated and does not have a standard to meet. Instead, people with PTSD can utilize a hand, a brush, or a pencil and allow the pain they are experiencing to come out. This process facilitates exiting the troubled waters of their minds.

PTSD promotes the impulse to withdraw, hide, and tamp down memories, instead of allowing those memories to be addressed. Visual art is not the only means of expression in PTSD patients. Poetry, music, and dance can also work well to express the pain, fear, and trauma of PTSD. Movement therapy is also a therapy field, as is music therapy. Poetry can be created and discussed with mental health practitioners. The words within poetry might offer insight into unique triggers and fears.

Ultimately, the goal of all art therapy modalities is personal expression. When the body and brain are given the freedom to express the terror, confusion, and grief so common to traumatic events, patients can release some of the power of PTSD. https://www.betterhelp.com/advice/ptsd/healing-from-ptsd-art-and-expression-as-a-treatment-modality/

**Music Therapy**
From:
https://www.percussionplay.com/music-as-medicine-ptsd-music-therapy/

"Music therapy was actually devised initially as a trauma response to aid the treatment of World War II veterans. Much of the research which has since surfaced identifies the therapeutic technique with the treatment of those suffering from post-traumatic stress as a result of experiences in warzones, natural disasters and physically violent confrontations. Inevitably, however, those with PTSD are not limited to people who have emerged from such circumstances: severe trauma of any nature can manifest in the development of the condition, and in addition to the groups mentioned above, minority groups, women and children are also likely to suffer from PTSD as a result of abuse."

"Research has demonstrated that people with PTSD respond particularly well to musical therapies. This is due, in part, to the relationships between stimuli provoked by music and the access to and post-processing of traumatic events. Music is uniquely designed to achieve this: non-threatening mediums such as music have often been seen to stimulate recollections of traumatic memories. These recollections can then be brought to the forefront of the mind in a controlled setting where the participant can experience being more empowered. That allows them to engage and interact with their emotionally traumatic memories in order to heal."

Essentially, the traumatic memory, during a flashback or nightmare, is frozen in the part of the brain which initially registered the original traumatic experience – making engaging with the memory, the feelings or emotions surrounding or associated with it, an incredibly difficult pathway to create in the brain. Music is proving to be useful in forging this pathway.

Another type of music therapy is group drumming sessions. Some done with combat veterans in Israel were recorded with digital cameras and sound which picked up patterns and observed changes in body language, verbal communication and external engagement among participants and the therapist. Open-ended in-depth interviews with the participants, and a self-report carried out by the therapist in charge also provided helpful data. Multiple symptomatic changes were noted as the sessions progressed: notably, the veterans experienced an increase in feelings of "openness, togetherness, belonging, sharing, closeness, connectedness and intimacy, as well as achieving a non-intimidating access to traumatic memories, facilitating an outlet for rage and regaining a sense of self-control." (Bensimon, Moshe et al. "Drumming through Trauma: Music Therapy with Post-Traumatic Soldiers." *The Arts in Psychotherapy*, vol. 35, 2008. pp. 24-48.) In other words, group drumming as a therapeutic technique proved to be hugely successful in many ways.

Personal testimonies from participants in the study confirmed such thinking. One participant noted: "All of the mutual crazy drumming created openness which enabled free talking about everything. Once you beat the drum, although you don't know anyone, it gives a feeling of togetherness which makes it possible for you to share everything with the group. It's as if you'll go naked in front of them. Yes! Exactly! As if they saw everything, so I can tell them all about myself. If I spoke about personal issues, it's only due to the group drumming which enabled us to open up. It brought us closer to each other when we hit the drums. I really connected myself with the group members. It's like working together. If something facilitated intimacy above all the instruments, it was the drums." (Bensimon, Moshe et al. "Drumming through Trauma: Music Therapy with Post-Traumatic Soldiers." *The Arts in Psychotherapy,* vol. 35, 2008. pp. 24-48.)

The facilitation of a genuine sense of interpersonal connection, belonging and fellowship is a primary aim in group therapies with PTSD sufferers. Therefore, the devising of innovative and effective techniques which allow for this sense of connectedness and openness to occur, even in the context of the avoidant nature of the condition, is vital to the success of such programs.

In the face of trauma, verbal communication with therapists can prove to be extremely difficult and sometimes impossible for those with PTSD. Using music as a neutral middle ground between patient and therapist is a valuable tool. This is from *Music as Medicine.* https://www.percussionplay.com/music-as-medicine-ptsd-music-therapy/

Research has shown that music therapy can provide:

- Nonverbal outlet for emotional expression
- Reduction in anxiety and stress
- Improvement in emotional state and mood
- Empowerment for the client
- Improved physiological changes (better blood pressure, heart rate, etc.)

- Opportunity for sharing and connecting with friends/loved ones
- Increased relaxation
- Safe place for self-expression
- Creative outlet

Music therapy is regularly used as a way to help manage stress and cope with difficult situations. Studies in neuroscience have suggested that music can help the brain rewire itself to learn new skills and/or reprogram old pathways into new ones. Music can't erase old memories, but it can possibly help to see them from a different perspective. (from https://imageryandmusic.com/music-therapy-and-ptsd/)

The following is from:
https://brainwavepowermusic.com/blogs/brainwave-power-music-s-articles/posts/using-music-to-treat-posttraumatic-stress-disorder-ptsd

Experts in the field have attributed the occurrence of PTSD to the overloading of the adrenaline response of the body during traumatic events, which in turn can cause a chain reaction of biochemical changes in the brain and the body. Hormones that involve the response to stress, fear, and danger all get affected, leading to a change in behavior of the affected person.

In addition, areas of the brain also become altered, specifically, the amygdala that is involved in the formation of emotional memories, as well as the hippocampus, which controls the ability to place memories in the right space and time context, as well as recalling memory. Studies have shown that music can trigger the brain to release chemicals to distract the body and mind from the pain. Music, as well as binaural beats and isochronic tones which augment the effects, reach the brain's auditory cortex, which causes the communication between the cortex and the sections of the brain that govern emotion, memory, and body control.

However, not just any music can work. Songs that have words, sung or spoken, can cause agitation when it's used for PTSD patients. Music and sounds that have low pitches are most effective, as well as music that is slow and has a steady beat. Although each patient may react differently to different songs, these kinds of songs have been proven to work best.

Music with binaural beats and isochronic tones have been shown to be even more potent in fighting off the effects of PTSD. This binaural beats track for PTSD is an example.
https://www.youtube.com/watch?v=6vrACw36z1E

"This music therapy track was made to give comfort and deep relaxation to those who are suffering from the disorder. We carefully embedded binaural beats that range from 0.20Hz to 10Hz, which are associated with the effects of the sleep state, the unconscious mind reaching out to gain better understanding and reflection, empathetic attainment, divine knowledge, inner being and personal growth, as well as trauma recovery, feeling blissful and being one with the universe. It is also a Spiritual Journey music accompaniment for those who seek the deeper essences of who we are. The binaural beat range also contains pain relief and sedative effects. As the carrier frequency of 136.1Hz resonates with the Earth, it will give you an overall sense of calming, centering, and is connected to the Heart chakra. May this music therapy track provide you with Love and Light."

From:
https://brainwavepowermusic.com/blogs/brainwave-power-music-s-articles/posts/using-music-to-treat-posttraumatic-stress-disorder-ptsd

Research scientist Adrienna Heinz of the National Center for Post-traumatic Stress Disorder claims that music therapy has the potential to help those struggling with PTSD. She adds, "More specifically, music therapy may be considered a resilience-enhancing intervention, as it can help trauma-exposed individuals harness their ability to recover elements of normality in their life following great adversity."

https://health.usnews.com/health-care/patient-advice/articles/2018-05-22/accessing-the-mental-health-benefits-of-music-therapy

Over the past twenty years, the field of neuroscience has grown exponentially and has contributed to advancing art therapy to the forefront of trauma-focused treatment today. Significant to the use of art therapy in trauma work is understanding the neurobiology of trauma, the biological study of the effects of trauma on the nervous system.

Advances in medical technology, such as brain imaging, now allow physicians, therapists, and scientists to literally see and understand what art therapists have known all along: creating, such as art-making, can change neural pathways in the brain; and that potentially changes the way one thinks and feels.

Art Therapy is a profession that facilitates psychic integration through the creative process and within the context of the therapeutic relationship. Conscious and unconscious mental activity, mind-body connectedness, the use of mental and visual imagery, bi-lateral stimulation, and communication between the limbic system and cerebral cortex functioning underscore and illuminate the healing benefits of art therapy — none of which could take place without the flexibility of neuronal processes, otherwise known as neuroplasticity (King, 2016).

Creative arts therapists know through creating — whether through art, music, poetry, or drama — that traumatic memory can be readily accessed in a way that is far less threatening than traditional verbal therapies. Traumatic memories are often stored in images and other sensations rather than in words or through verbalization, and many art therapists have observed how making art helps in releasing traumatic memories that were previously inaccessible.

from:
https://psychcentral.com/ptsd/art-therapy-for-trauma

Recent developments in neuroscience have provided information about areas of the brain responsible for the verbal processing of traumatic events. Brain imaging illustrates that for many, when recounting a traumatic event, the Broca's area (language) of the brain shuts down, and at the same time, the amygdala becomes aroused (Tripp, 2007). Right brain activation through art media allows for less reliance on the verbal languages area of the brain, which provides some substantiation for why nonverbal therapies like art therapy might be more effective when working with trauma (Klorer, 2005).

**Theater**

The following is from this article used with permission: https://www.psychotherapynetworker.org/article/theater-therapy/

First Gulf War-era veteran and professional actor, Stephan Wolfert, who is now testing a PTSD intervention that for decades has been pairing classical theater training with the science of trauma. The following is from the Psychotherapy Networker blog.

Wolfert's autobiographical one-man play, *Cry Havoc*, was a highlight of the 2018 Psychotherapy Networker Symposium, and his acting intervention, De-Cruit, which is currently being evaluated at New York University and is showing impressive early results. A novel combination of mindfulness, narrative therapy, resilience training, exposure, psychodynamics, community building, and the plays of Shakespeare, along with De-Cruit, teaches vets how to take to the stage to disentangle themselves from their soldier training, process their experience at war, and connect with the very different reality of being home. Wolfert is interviewed below.

***Ryan Howes, PhD, ABPP****, a psychologist, writer, musician, and clinical professor at Fuller Graduate School of Psychology in Pasadena, California,* is the interviewer RH.

**RH:** Plenty of modern theater takes on trauma. Why, in this day and age, are you championing Shakespeare as a conduit to healing?

**Wolfert:** Because it worked for me. As I say in *Cry Havoc*, I didn't realize, after a friend of mine was killed at a military training center, that I was having a psychotic break. Drunk somewhere in Montana, I ended up hopping off a train and wandering into a performance of *Richard the Third*. If you know the play, you know Richard was a veteran of war. I didn't know that at the time. All I remember is a guy in uniform walking out on stage, looking me directly in the eye, and saying, "The war is over, and there is a time of peace, and it's fantastic. Everyone's happy, except me, because I feel deformed, because I don't fit in, because I'm not attractive. I don't even like peace."

That was it. I left the army and went to graduate school for acting. Then I started reading Shakespeare and found that he wrote about and, in fact, was surrounded by veterans. When he was writing *Hamlet, Henry the Fifth, As You Like It*, and *Julius Caesar*, England was in two wars: a conventional war with Spain, with cold war components to it—similar to what I went through—and the Nine Years' War with Ireland, which was mostly guerrilla warfare. They have ballads in England about men who came home from Ireland but never "fully" returned.

**RH:** You talk about the need for a "de-cruiting" process for soldiers like you who've been "wired for war." What do you mean by this?

**Wolfert:** It means the military rewires the central nervous system and creates automatic, mind–body responses to war stimuli. For example, outside the military, if you hear bullets flying over your head, you may instinctively duck and take cover, but that instinct is rewired in soldiers, so that we respond to it with violence instead. In the infantry, when we hear a rifle shot, we immediately locate the general vicinity it came from and return fire in that direction.

In basic training, they drill these automatic responses into us, but when we get out, we don't have eight weeks of basic *untraining*. We don't learn how to leave those responses behind.

**RH:** Are you contending that a focus on classical acting training helps with this rewiring?

**Wolfert:** Yes, I am. And our scientific evaluation is proving it. The basic tenets of theater are medicine. Yvette Nolan talks about this in her book *Medicine Shows*. Further, classical actor training contains some of the most successful components of therapy, such as camaraderie in a creative, expressive, and healing environment; mindfulness and raising self-awareness without judgment; and Shakespeare's heightened language, written in our natural human rhythm, which provides a certain aesthetic distance from our own experience, making us feel safer to disclose. These components are similar to those the military used to wire us for war, so I'm using them to rewire from war.

**RH:** In the case of PTSD sufferers, you might be taking them out of the fight-or-flight state they experience every day?

**Wolfert:** Being in front of an audience feels like life or death. Just like Shakespeare's characters, we think something, or we feel something, and we speak it out loud to a room of strangers. There's a power in that, releasing our stories, and having that experience rewarded and reinforced by a group or an audience. Then, when we've survived that heightened experience of sharing our trauma out loud, we've not only taught our body that we'll survive reliving that event, but we've also begun to rewire the brain out of that continual state of fight or flight.

**RH:** What does it do for veterans, casting aside social buffers like that?

**Wolfert:** Once we're in that place, we begin really expressing ourselves. The three questions I'm always asking them are: What do you feel? Where in your body do you feel it? And when else have you felt that way? This helps them start to track their habits and default modes. Going deeper, I do writing prompts aimed at taking on significant events in our life. Like Bessel Van Der Kolk talks about in *The Body Keeps the Score*, instead of merely repeating our own reel, the act of writing it out changes things.

**RH:** So, I'm going to better see my trauma simply by turning it into a narrative?

**Wolfert:** And by getting it on paper. Sometimes when we do longer programs, we have vets read each other's works, so they can also hear it.

**RH:** What you're doing sounds a lot like exposure, but with a twist of built-in relaxation and detachment. What's your message for therapists about the power of a theater intervention like this?

**Wolfert:** I always encourage therapists to bring art into their practice. And it can be in whatever form they're most passionate about. Obviously, I'm partial to theater because it works for me. But I also feel that theater has a special power because it connects us with everything — our bodies and our emotions.

I've worked with Twyla Tharp, and she believes it's all about the body. I agree with her, but I feel the voice is part of the body. If we can bring theater to it, then we have an actor and an audience. And ultimately, what is therapy but an actor and an audience? From: *An Unusual Program is Helping Vets Rewire from War* by Ryan Howes. Source:
https://www.psychotherapynetworker.org/article/theater-therapy/

Theater-based therapeutic programs can help people of all ages to feel seen and heard, to raise awareness for change, and to explore and respond to challenging material onstage in a safe and supportive environment. As noted in a profile in STAT News, of Van Der Kolk's theater-based program, "The students experience the same sort of threatening situations in the scenes, but because they are not in real danger, they are able to react in new ways.
https://www.statnews.com/2016/08/23/theater-trauma-teenagers/

The key is that the person with PTSD has well known responses to situations, but in theater you get to explore and experiment with new options. Playing out those new options in a different character (not their own identity) gives them flexibility and empowers them in new ways. Van Der Kolk relates the story of his son who in theater took on different ways of being that worked for him and he felt good enough that he adopted a new way of being and was no longer stuck and unhappy.

While there is no one-size-fits-all approach to trauma recovery, some survivors find theatrical expression to be more valuable than traditional talk therapy. In an essay, Canadian social worker and activist, Vikki Reynolds, recounts a story of a young Guatemalan survivor she worked with, who participated in a session of Theater of the Oppressed, a "form of popular community-based education that uses theater for social change," created by Brazilian Nobel Peace Prize nominee Agusto Boal. When Reynolds asked the young person how that session compared to talk therapy, she said that it was worth "over a hundred" traditional talk therapy sessions.
https://mentalhealthcampaign.org/2019/09/03/therapy-on-stage-reclaiming-power-healing-trauma-through-theater-and-the-expressive-arts/

Between the time I wrote the above and editing it, I did some musical theater myself. I took a class called Veteran Storytelling and it turned out to be an acting class. I liked the teacher and decided to stay. I learned a lot in that class and was encouraged to audition for two shows at the Seattle Repertory Theater. The first one was a workshop of a new show they were creating. I was in the ensemble singing. Because it was a workshop lasting only three weeks, and we had our books in front of us as we sang, it seemed easy. The second audition was a Shakespeare show called the Tempest. I was given a part in the ensemble again. There was a lot to learn in the many songs, the nuances of the songs and all the choreography. I was overwhelmed with so much to learn and remember, as well as perform. I practiced a lot even at home, not trusting my ability to remember it all with the sequences. My teacher, was an actor. The first day of class, I said, "I know nothing about acting! I only know how to be authentic." He responded by saying: "Acting is being authentic!" I did not believe that until the day of our dress rehearsal for The Tempest when I was on stage in costume in the role of earth spirit. I was responding to everything that happened in every scene I was in, and it was all authentically me. I felt so many feelings throughout the show and they were all authentic. I finally understood what he meant. Acting is being authentic, that is what makes it work.

If you have a chance to be part of a theater group, I encourage you to do it. Not only do you get to experience yourself differently and try out new things but you will be part of a community of others who, like you are experimenting, expressing and perhaps even healing as well.

## 8. MARTIAL ARTS

University of South Florida professor, Alison Willing, says costly intense therapy and medication has a low success rate. This is why she's studying the effects of Jiu Jitsu on PTSD. She conducted a study on the possible respite of PTSD through the practice of Brazilian Jiu Jitsu, as well as traditional exercise. Willing said the study came together when many veterans who train at Tampa Jiu Jitsu, a local gym, reported the benefits they saw from the martial art for their PTSD symptoms. The study is designed to alleviate the symptoms of PTSD, rather than attempting to cure the disorder, and for some veterans it is proving to be their best option to eliminate sleepless nights.

"The effects of this first study were so dramatic. The PTSD scores on all of the valid scales were getting so much better to the point where you don't usually see with traditional PTSD therapies," explains Alison Willing, a professor at the USF Center of Aging and Brain Repair. Jacob's headaches and sleepless nights have pretty much gone away. Read article: (from https://www.ptsduk.org/martial-arts/)

Martial arts allow you to understand and develop a good relationship with power, helps you express emotions, helps to practice self-care, helps set and maintain boundaries, can help you relax, and can also help with disassociation by reconnecting the body and mind with repetitive movements.

It is thought that the concentration, discipline and training of martial arts, have been found to aid the healing process for some PTSD sufferers. "I can't tell you what it is exactly about this discipline that pulls me back from the edge. All I know is that at first, when my instructor's hands went around my throat in a chokehold, I would be flung straight into the claws of a panic attack. Now… well, not so much," notes Sonia Lena. "I've been dealing with C-PTSD for a very long time now. It's a constant, unwelcome companion, but the intensity of it comes in waves; sometimes the symptoms are fierce, other times they're more manageable. And sometimes it almost feels like they're gone. My panic attacks are less frequent and more manageable. Generally, I can wake up from a nightmare and not spend the rest of the night wide awake. Generally, I can have a flashback and not throw up from the shock of it. Not all the time, but enough that it counts."

Mixed martial arts (MMA) – a sport which incorporates elements of boxing, kickboxing and wrestling – is another form of martial arts which has been found to help when it comes to addressing PTSD.

More specifically, hapkido is a non-competitive form of martial arts, promoting patience, discipline and internal harmony and so "there's no ego involved" said Mike Fournier an instructor and Founder of East Coast Combat Hapkido. "When done properly, it helps to re-center and refocus yourself."

Whether it is the physical or mental aspect of martial arts which is most effective for those with PTSD is likely to depend on the individual, but one thing is for sure, it is working.
from https://www.ptsduk.org/martial-arts/

Aikido is a proven and tested martial art that is practiced by millions of people worldwide, you can start at any age, young or old, male or female, no experience in martial arts and no need for size or physical strength. Aikido was created by Morihei Ueshiba who is widely considered to be The World's Greatest Martial Artist. The Founder or Sensei (Great Teacher) was a military man who went undefeated after facing every challenge from boxers, Karatekas, Wrestlers, Kickboxers,

Judokas, Jujutsu, Kenjutsu, Sumo & Kendo experts. Unlike other martial arts that rely heavenly on physical strength and size, Aikido teaches students to use the size, strength, speed and aggression of their attacker against them. In Aikido you learn to blend simultaneously with the attack and put the opponent under your control and in an off-balance position, then execute the appropriate Aikido technique. Aikido's curriculum includes: Atemi (strikes with your fist, hands, fingers, palms, forearms, elbows, knees, shins, feet, etc to the opponent's eyes, throat, temples, nose, chin, jaw, solar plexus, ribs, stomach, groin, knees, shins, toes, spine etc); Throwing & Takedowns (Throwing opponents which requires no physical strength or size whatsoever); Chokes & Strangles (Chokes that attack the blood, air & nerve pathways to the brain); Weapons Training & Weapons Disarming (You learn to use The Mighty Katana or Samurai Sword, The Jo or Samurai Quarter Staff, Tanto or Samurai Battle Knife); Multiple Attacker Defense (Defense against two or more opponents); Meditation & Emotional Control (Learn to control the mind & emotions no matter how stressful the situation); and Self-Respect & Honor (young people learn to not only respect themselves but also to respect others, which is important in this world). Unlike other martial arts, Aikido has no competition because the Martial Way focuses on real life self-defense and survival skills (in fact, what works in fighting quite often fail in real life survival situations). Aikido is not a sport in any way but rather it's a Way of Life. The Founder or O Sensei was a genius in not only Military Combat but also in The Strategy of Life... meaning what you learn in Aikido is not only for Combat & Self Defense, rather The Aikido Way carries over organically into everyday life just as the Founder intended. This is why Aikido is very popular with the armed forces, police and leaders in all walks of life worldwide. https://www.youtube.com/watch?v=R_nSKo34S5Y

I wanted to chime in here since it seems relevant and fitting at this point. I began studying Aikido in 2000 after going through many devastating losses. My thinking and responses were sluggish, I thought it was crazy to be sixty-years-old and signing up for a martial art, but felt strongly from my own inner wisdom that was what I needed to do right then. I stayed with it for years until the dojo closed due to the Covid-19 crisis. I made it all the way to Sandan, third degree black belt.

It helped me tremendously over the years and especially when my own PTSD was triggered. The very first time I was studying the choke hold and someone put one on me. I was frozen and could not breathe, speak or move. My sensei, Pam Cooper, gently told me what to do: with one arm, simply pull the opponent's elbow outward so I could breathe. I realized that choke holds were going to be triggering me and went to a friend who did cranio-sacral energy work. After she worked on me and we released my old birth trauma, I had no more trouble doing or experiencing chokeholds.

When previously discussing triggers, I shared mine from when the back door of the dojo was open. This time, I use the same experience to discuss a flashback.

I walked over to the door and looked out and BAM! I was in a flashback, staring at a busy street in Vietnam. My knees nearly giving out, I turned back into the dojo, trying to find my breath. I told my sensei, and she said to wait until it passed to get back on the mat.

I truly believe for me in Aikido that the focus, the concentration, the need to be in the moment and the movement all helped me restore balance in my mind and body. Aikido is all about movement. Number one, is move to a safe place. The angle in relation to the attacker is essential in finding a safe place. I had been learning that lesson for years and it was probably twelve or more years into it when a visitor from another dojo in another state came to do Aikido with us for a week. The guy was well trained, fast and aggressive. He was doing *irimi nage* (entering throw) with me. I remembered learning to go right into his center and stay glued there. It saved me. He was not able to throw me. I like being on the 45° and to apply *irimi nage* myself.

In the beginning, I was very clumsy and slow but as I came out of my depression and began to feel more confident, I felt better. Another important thing about Aikido is that it is based on a health system. As we do Aikido, our movements are stimulating the flow of energy through our bodies. That energy flow is important to health and balance. Any day that I did not feel well and was considering not going to training, I would go anyway and usually before the class was over, I felt better simply because I was moving good energy through my body. Aikido is not an aggressive martial art like Jiu Jitsu. It started out that way in Jiu Jitsu which Morihei Ueshiba taught to the Japanese Army, but after the war, he became more self-reflective, spiritual, and created the new system called the Way of Harmony, or Aikido, based on the same principles but less aggressive and hurtful. In Jiu Jitsu you can literally break bones. In Aikido we protect ourselves and our attacker. Because Aikido is fun, it is healing to do. Even when we get to the level where we attack and receive attacks from knife, sword, Bo, and even bat. Again, it is important to immediately move to a safe place when we are being attacked and then apply whatever technique is appropriate for where we are. For black belt we learn to deal with four attackers at once and not get trapped. At the time I signed up for Aikido, I had no idea it could help me in so many ways, but it did and I highly recommend it for anyone young or old who needs to move, have fun, learn self-protection and feel good. I recommend that if you do choose to do Aikido, look for a dojo and teacher that practices in a way that fits for you. I did that and decided on the Aikido of West Seattle and it was the best choice for me.

The following is from:
http://www.searchofpeace.com/blog/2015/05/27/osensei-a-war-veteran-with-ptsd/

Before the war, Morihei was recognized as a master of most styles of martial arts in Japan at the time. After the war ended, Morihei put these considerable martial arts skills aside and eventually turned to the calming, nonviolent world of farming. It was also during this time that he joined the Ōmoto-kyō movement. During this period, he further developed martial arts mastery. His commitment to Budo, his indomitable will, and his deep spirituality enabled him to resolve his own issues and find a way through his PTSD. He was able to see that there was a possible path for him to peace through the proper application of martial disciplines. His strength of character and morality informed the development of a way to bring this path to a world committed to warfare and the universal suffering of PTSD.

His search started with Daito-Ryu Aikijujutsu. Within this style, he organized his own form of aikijujutsu, which he called Aiki Bujutsu. He later used this as a starting point from which to create his own martial art, which he renamed Aiki Budo. Morihei incorporated his mastery of other ancient martial arts, adding elements of many of these, including swordsmanship and kito-ryu ju jutsu, and blended these with many techniques of his own. Emphasis was always placed on using ki, or centered inner power, to increase a person's strength. The final iteration of his martial art he named ai-ki-do, "way to a unified spirit." Throughout this path of developing Aikido, it appears that he was always striving for a way to more peacefully resolve conflict. In keeping with this, I believe that O Sensei intends the practice of Aikido technique to be a pathway for developing that calm, centered, internal peace which we can then take into the world as a way to promote peace.

I believe that every great philosophy, every significant idea which has played a role in the development of humanity, of human nature, has come from a deep, very personal place in one individual who sees the positive effect this will have on the world and has the strength of character, commitment, perseverance and entrepreneurial drive to bring it to the world. Morihei Ueshiba, O Sensei, found this inner well-source and had that drive.

O Sensei has said that Aikido is a way to bring peace to the world, but one cannot bring peace to the world without first achieving peace within oneself. However, to only achieve inner peace, without then offering this pathway to the world, is not at all in keeping with the life and the teachings he expressed through his Aikido. We do not have to be combat veterans to achieve, or even understand, the centered, calm, peaceful state which can come from the proper practice of Aikido. Likewise, we do not have to have an advanced rank to make a sincere effort to expand that inner peace, to offer it to those suffering from trauma, to bring it to organizations involved in striving for peace, to make our own sincere effort to bring peace to the world.
from:

http://www.searchofpeace.com/blog/2015/05/27/osensei-a-war-veteran-with-ptsd/

## 9. ROWING

I met a Vietnam Veteran named Steve Wells from Evergreen Rowing years ago. He talked about the calming nature of rowing and the strength and focus required to do it well. I had always been afraid of the water and was not a good swimmer, so I had avoided water activities, but was intrigued about rowing.

Steve took me out in a Maas Aero single and just had me sit in it and feel what it was like for him to move the boat back and forth at the edge of the beach. For my next step, which came sooner than I might have thought I was ready for, he set me in the boat by myself and rowed alongside me in his own boat. He showed me what to do and talked me through it. I felt safe enough to sign up for a twelve-week rowing class at a club nearby. We learned in Wherries, which are the safest boats to train in, as they are like big tubs and do not tip over. I did pretty well but still was not sure it was something I wanted to stick with.

I learned about a camp in Vermont called Craftsbury where they offered programs on rowing, with the in-between times filled with yoga. It sounded perfect, and I signed up for the five-day course. We had three rowing sessions a day and they videotaped us individually so we could watch later with coaches and learn from it. It was excellent. The first day out, I was in a flyweight by Maas, which was a step up from the Aero I had been using. The flyweight was much skinnier and much more tippy. The coach helped me get over my fear of the water and flipping; that was huge for me and made it so much easier to relax my body and learn to row better. I learned a lot about water and boat safety, rowing techniques, types of oars, and the boats themselves. I also met some wonderful people and did one race at the very end. I could tell racing was not my thing but it was a good experience to have. I also got to be in a team boat once and learned quickly how my small size makes it difficult to keep up with bigger faster rowers. I am glad I did it and really liked feeling the power of a team rowing together and how fast they go.

Wherever you live, if you are by rivers or big lakes, you may be able to find a rowing club where they teach rowing. Many clubs offer a "learn to row" day or class in the spring. If you have any interest or believe it could help you relax and enjoy nature, then try it out. You will know relatively quickly if it is right for you. Getting into a club, meeting the people and learning in a four or eight team boat is easier than learning to row a single. In a team boat with four people rowing, you have one oar and learn the technique for that crew and boat. Hopefully, you have repeated experiences doing that and feel more confident. If interested, please go to YouTube and look for either men or women, depending on your gender, rowing in fours or eights. That will show you what it looks like. You can do the same for singles or doubles. In a single or a double, or a quad, you are sculling and have two oars. It is very different than rowing a four or eight with only one oar. Rowing is not for everyone but it is a fun and challenging sport and was helpful to me. I like the feeling of gliding across the water, the peacefulness of it and being able to see eagles and blue herons. When I was part of the rowing club on the Duwamish River as a coxswain, I loved seeing Mount Rainier and seeing the salmon jump, when in season, and the osprey flying. If you happen to be small like me, or find that the rowing itself is too much of a challenge, being a coxswain for a team boat is another wonderful possibility.

## 10. CEREMONY

Ceremony is a healing adventure and Welcome Home for the Whole Warrior. Called the Rite of Return, it is a rite of passage for prior service-members seeking to answer the soul's call for deep healing in the wilderness, in order to lay down what no longer serves you and step into who you are truly called to be after military service. Separated from society, in solidarity and solitude, cross the threshold as a Whole Warrior to answer *Who Am I? What's My Purpose? Where do I Belong?*

This ancient, cross-cultural ceremony has proven to drastically reduce the symptoms of post-traumatic stress, compassion fatigue, moral injury, and suicidal ideation by embracing the wholeness of our human experience and true nature. Veteran Rites has continued evaluation in partnership with Mark Van Ryzin of the University of Oregon Research Institute. It is a bare-bones, universal container that deeply honors any warrior's unique abilities, values, belief system, culture, and identity so they can do what is theirs to do and sing the songs that are theirs to sing.

The eleven- day ceremony is held in the wilderness of Eastern Washington with trained veteran and non-veteran guides. Participants experience time in community with other vets, four days of solo time, fasting in the wilderness, and a marked return, where their stories are shared and witnessed in a "council of elders." This return marks the beginning of a veteran's process of incorporating that which they have gained and learned during their time in service and explored in the context of time alone in the wilderness, so they may bring their gifts home, and be able to participate more fully in service to their families and their community. Initiates will be supported throughout their incorporation year by Veteran Rites and the circle of whole warriors as they claim their truth.

The Rite of Return is available to current and prior military service members, spouses, partners, Gold Star parents and eighteen + dependent survivors of veteran suicide. Veteran Rites will work with every warrior called to the land to fully prepare physically, mentally, and spiritually for their Rite of Return journey and address unique barriers and conditions that may prevent participation.

For more information: email Executive Director and Seabee Veteran (OIF) Ryan Mielcarek at council@veteranrites.org or call (206) 228-5466 and you can sit for a spell, share stories, and see if this ceremony (not program) is right for you.

I did my own ceremony in September of 2020 and was the oldest veteran to do so. I was eighty at the time. I believe I may have been the first Vietnam Veteran to go through the process. What I can tell you about my own experience is that I had been hearing about it for many months from Ryan and was very interested in doing it, but had to wait until I dealt with some health issues before going. That time came the end of August 2020 which allowed me to be part of the group going out in September. They provided me with a list of all that I would need to bring and be prepared for and I added what I knew I would personally need beyond that. The process of gathering all that and packing took about two weeks or more.

There were two books to read to prepare and I started early to read those. One was *The Roaring of the Sacred River* by Steven Foster and Meredith Little and the other was *The Four Shields: The Initiatory Seasons of Human Nature* by the same authors.

I shared the drive up with another veteran I knew. We were greeted, given instructions and support to find a place for our tent and personal gear. Because of my age and physical limitations, two of the guys set up my tent for me. Veteran Rites provided a large bag of snack foods, fruit and other goodies and there were coolers for our perishable items. I had dehydrated some of my own grass-fed beef jerky, fruit and veggies. I was also given a Veteran Rites sweat shirt and t-shirt and later some rope and a ground cloth for my vision fast.

We met in circle for several hours and got to know each other, shared our stories, why we were there, and any other prompts given to us. It was deep, authentic, emotional, and supportive. We did that many times for different purposes over the first four days and after our vision fasts.

We were first guided to go out on the land and find our own place for the vision fast and then took our four gallons of water there. Fortunately, I had help to do that as well. We were taught things we needed to know like how to set up our tarp for protection from the sun and elements, what to look for and how to stay safe during our vision fast.

Those of us veterans who were doing ceremony were in a separate space than the staff so we had meal times together and we were on our own for breakfast, lunch and dinner for the days before our vision fast. I could tell that my body was preparing for the fast by eating less and less each day.

Because one of our group was a woman veteran from Alaska who had brought a bunch of fresh salmon with her, we feasted on that salmon and some other things for our last dinner together before our vision fast. I helped prepare some of the condiments that went with our dinner and everyone helped set it up and clean up.

The morning we were to leave for our four days of solo time and vision fast, we all awoke well before dawn. Whether it be due to the excitement or anticipation, I was not sure, but that morning there seemed to be a spring in our step as we carried our gear out to the area set up for our departure. Once we are all gathered, and our packs ready, we held a small ceremony preparing us for what lay ahead. With that, we crossed the threshold and set off alone, each on our own little journey.

I had attended Long Dance for twenty years and was excited and happy to be out on the land for four days to commune with and be surrounded by nature and the Divine. I had a dear friend who was also a Long Dancer and who was consciously dying from cancer, and I dedicated the fast to her in support of her process unfolding as she desired.

I was already turning inward, even as I focused on the physical journey down the hill and then on to where I would set up my space for the vision fast. I had my walking stick from Long Dance which helped me stabilize when I encountered hidden rocks.

When I arrived at my spot and had stowed aside my bags and gear, I began to search out a place to set up a sacred altar which could be the center of my vision fast space. There were a lot of trees in that space, but one of them immediately caught my eye, as it seemed taller than the rest — the bark at its base blackened by a fire in its distant past. A good sign that it, like me, had survived some troubling times. There was a small area at the base of that tree that was perfect for what I needed.

I used some rocks that I had brought, along with some pine cones and moss I collected from nearby, to create the focal point that I needed.

Truly the Divine One was everywhere, under and around me, but the sacred altar space was as precious to me as it might be in church. I had brought a three-legged camp chair and put it in front of my altar. I set up the ground cloth that Ryan loaned me and put the tarp over it and then had a place to sit, lie down, put my personal items, etc. The four gallons of water were at the base of another tree. I put my sleeping pad and sleeping bag out in the open field nearby. I always like to see the sky when sleeping on the land. Even when I have a tent, I like to leave the top open to see the sky and only put on the rain fly when absolutely necessary. I was sure I would be happy out in the field under the open sky and I was. At night, I could see the moon, stars, and even the planets Saturn and Jupiter.

After I had everything set up, I took a walk around the area to see what was there. I had specifically chosen that area because there were a lot of dead and fallen trees. Since I knew I was in the West and focused on grieving, it seemed appropriate for me to be surrounded by dead trees to support my grief. I also found an area further away that had a fallen tree I could sit on. When I was sitting on that tree, I saw what looked like miniature squirrels with a yellow and black stripe down their back. Those miniature squirrels were fast in every movement they made. They were intriguing to me.

I spent a lot of my time there grieving with those fallen trees, but also just getting the needed rest my body and soul seemed to need. I was careful to drink my water with electrolytes. I spent some time each day walking with my walking stick. The area was full of hidden rocks not visible until I was on top of them and the walking stick helped me stabilize and not fall. I made sure to find time in each day for heartfelt prayers and singing the songs I had learned from the Long Dance. In fact, I learned that singing the songs helped me connect to my grief.

Because of my purpose and grief, I was in the West Shield much of my time out there and then moved to the North. My personal goal was to get to the East and with guidance from the Divine, open up my vision for what is ahead for me in my life. In the morning of the fourth day of my vision fast, the winds had changed and were blowing cooler air. I wondered if it was the connection to the North Shield? I also noted that the smoke we had seen in the distance seemed to be moving closer to where we were. I soon had to put on the sweatshirt and then a fleece jacket for warmth. Then even later, I was leaning back on my rolled-up sleeping bag meditating and asking for my vision, when one of the staff came to me. I am not sure how long he was there because I was deep in my meditation — but I eventually heard him saying that we needed to move. I was not sure what that meant because I had been moving every day. As I brought my awareness back to the present and what he was saying, I realized that he wanted me to break camp and move back up the hill. The shift in winds and smoke made it more dangerous for our group and so we were moving to a different camp. I was unhappy and upset by this disruption because I was deep into what I was there for and did not want to abort the process. While I was ever so glad the staff was keeping us safe, at the same time, I was frustrated by having to leave and interrupt my process. We did have to move to another camp and it took many hours to pack up the entire camp and all the tents, clothing, food, gear, etc.

The tail end of the vision fast experience was to tell our stories and process our experiences. It was amazing to hear everyone's story and how different they all were, but so powerful and so uniquely them. Each story reflected that person and their experiences and the elders listened and mirrored back the essence of each one. They were all deep, intense, informative, and personal. I was honored to be with each of the veterans in our group, get to know them and feel connected to them and their stories.

I highly recommend doing the ceremony/vision fast with Veteran Rites for your own purposes, whether it is to feel connected to yourself, the land, your purpose, your own spirituality, your body, your family, whatever it is, you will be guided and supported well. Meeting the challenge in front of you in an authentic supportive community of veterans is priceless and will serve you as you move forward in your life.

# Chapter 12
# ATTITUDES AND BELIEFS

I believe PTSD can be healed. That does not mean that you will never again get triggered or feel anxious, rather it means that those symptoms of PTSD will only surface from time to time and never again dominate your daily life. Because you have gone through therapies of some type, you have the strength and skills to deal with whatever comes up. You may have been incapacitated by all the symptoms of PTSD before, but now you are in charge of your life and have an abundance of skills, resources and confidence to deal with any that resurface. You have taken PTSD seriously, gone through processes to work through and heal the trauma. You are no longer at the mercy of triggers that come up and you are mainly symptom free.

It seems to me that many therapists, programs and even the VA, do not believe what I wrote above. Either because they do not know how to heal PTSD or they do not have the resources to bring about the healing. The VA and many programs and therapists are focused on decreasing symptoms, because that is the most important metric for receiving an insurance payment. Decreasing your symptoms can be a relief, but it is not dealing with the actual trauma and healing it. You have a right to have help to put it all behind you so that you don't have to deal with it all of your life. The experiences will always be there because it happened to you and you know it, but it need not plague you once you have faced and dealt with the trauma.

Your attitude toward your PTSD and healing it, and the attitude of those around you, will have an impact on you and your therapy. If your attitude is negative toward yourself, your condition, and your ability to heal it, that will interfere with your achievement of success. If those around you do not trust you, believe what you say, or support you the way you need to be supported, that will interfere with your success in getting where you need to be. If the therapist or other helpers discount what you say, or the impact of your traumatic experiences, that too will interfere with your success to move through the process to heal. **You can heal**! To do that, you need to believe you can and trust yourself to do the work needed to heal from your trauma. You also need a good therapist that you trust, who is skilled at healing PTSD, and has a number of tools and techniques at his/her disposal to use in helping you heal. Having many tools is important. A therapist who only has one way to work in therapy, one method, will not be helpful. You also need a support system of people who will not undermine you or your process of healing. You need people who genuinely care about you and getting you back to the best you can be. Trauma changes people deeply and you will need to go through those same depths to restore and heal yourself so that you are stronger, clearer and better in every way than before the trauma. You are forever changed but it need not be in a negative way. There are PTSD support groups and there are groups for veterans, e.g., Veteran Rites Circle of Return which you can find on www.veteranrites.org,
https://vets4warriors.com,
https://www.veteranshealthlibrary.va.gov/142,UG4350_VA

Years ago, I had a consultant/trainer who worked with babies that had traumatic births. He showed me his technique for dealing with them and told me that those children grew up to have a stronger character than children who had easy births. He described their resiliency after being traumatized and helpless. Going through his therapy to heal the trauma built new abilities and character. You too can heal from the traumatic experiences and build a new you with new skills, abilities and character.

I truly believe healing trauma in a group is better than one-to-one because your group members can reflect back to you what they perceive, support you in between sessions, and be there for you when you need someone to talk with. The therapy I did while working as a nurse psychotherapist was individual with each person, one at a time within the group. When working with that one person, others are affected by what they see, hear and feel. They are watching, listening and having their own experiences. Their responses are from their own life and perspective. Once the focus on the one individual has been completed, the other group members are able to speak up and share what they experienced from what they saw, heard and felt, which often leads to them doing their own work piece on what was stimulated. Because there are established ground rules, each person knows how to respond in appropriate ways and to get the focus and attention they need for what is emerging from them. Also, in a group setting you can easily do psychodramas that include others. Everyone gets something out of each process and experience.

In a group you get to talk to your younger self or the self that endured the trauma, either using another group member to help, or projecting that part of you onto a pillow. All these active methods are therapeutic and helpful not only to you, but maybe your other group members. Everyone benefits from the work each of you do in front of each other. When the therapist is working with someone else, you benefit by seeing and hearing what is taking place and applying it to you or your situation. It will not always apply to you directly, but you can learn from it. You learn a lot about parenting by how the therapist responds to the child aspect of anyone in the group. There are many different scenarios that are brought in by group members from their family life, and when the therapist is directly talking to a child or even a parent. Much of that can translate into your own life as a parent.

The following is from information about PTSD online from WebMD.

PTSD therapy has three main goals:

- Improve your symptoms
- Teach you skills to deal with it
- Restore your self-esteem

***Note**: it is *not* a goal in this list to heal the trauma that caused the PTSD. From: https://www.webmd.com/mental-health/what-are-treatments-for-posttraumatic-stress-disorder#1

Most PTSD therapies fall under the umbrella of cognitive behavioral therapy (CBT). The idea is to change the thought patterns that are disturbing your life. This might happen through talking about your trauma or concentrating on where your fears come from.

**Cognitive Processing Therapy**

CPT is a twelve-week course of treatment, with weekly sessions of 60-90 minutes.

At first, you will talk about the traumatic event with your therapist and how your thoughts about it have affected your life. Then you will write in detail about what happened. This process helps you examine how you think about your trauma and figure out new ways to live with it.

For example, maybe you have been blaming yourself for something. Your therapist will help you take into account all the things that were beyond your control, so you can move forward, understanding and accepting that, deep down, it was not your fault, despite things you did or did not do.

**Prolonged Exposure Therapy**

If you have been avoiding things that remind you of the traumatic event, PE will help you confront them. It involves eight to fifteen sessions, usually ninety minutes each.

Early on in treatment, your therapist will teach you breathing techniques to ease your anxiety when you think about what happened. Later, you'll make a list of the things you've been avoiding and learn how to face them, one by one. In another session, you will recount the traumatic experience to your therapist, then go home and listen to a recording of yourself. Doing this as homework over time may help ease your symptoms.

Once you've learned self-calming techniques, you and your therapist will create a hierarchy of fears. You'll start with things you find slightly scary and progress to more intense fears — possibly those related to the trauma you experienced. You won't progress to the next level on your hierarchy until you and your therapist are satisfied you can handle each one.

Over several months of treatment, you and your therapist will work together to help you face your fears, allowing you to practice new coping skills. You'll learn that your thoughts and memories related to the trauma aren't actually dangerous and don't need to be avoided.

If during your therapy on exposure to the trauma your distress goes up, you can bring it down using EFT. You can do this for yourself if the therapist does not know it and then you can educate the therapist. More details page 241.

**Eye Movement Desensitization and Reprocessing**

With EMDR, you are in charge of the pace because you will focus on some aspect of the trauma and your inner guidance will take over to allow the memories to flow so you can see and feel for yourself what took place.

You will be focused on the therapist's hands as he/she moves them back and forth, following the movement with your eyes. The therapist may tap on your knees in an alternating pattern, or even make a sound on your right side, then your left.

There is a point at which something different happens and it may be something you thought of, or was created magically inside of you. Once that happens, everything changes. It is as if a switch flipped from negative to positive and you are feeling stronger and more fully resourced. To me, this is the magic of EMDR.

How many sessions are needed depends on your level of trauma. If, during EMDR, your stress level goes past five on a one to ten scale, it is useful to use EFT to bring it down to 0 before proceeding.

A 2018 review Trusted Source of research found that when provided by an experienced therapist, EMDR has the ability to reduce many symptoms of PTSD, including anxiety, depression, fatigue, and paranoid thought patterns. It's a low-cost therapy, has few if any side effects, and is recommended by the World Health Organization (WHO) for treatment of PTSD.

**Stress Inoculation Training**
SIT is a type of CBT. You can do it by yourself or in a group. You will not have to go into detail about what happened. The focus is more on changing how you deal with the stress from the event.

You might learn massage and breathing techniques and other ways to stop negative thoughts by relaxing your mind and body. After about three months, you should have the skills to release the added stress from your life.

**Medications**
The brains of people with PTSD process "threats" differently, in part because the balance of chemicals called neurotransmitters are out of balance. They have an easily triggered "fight or flight" response, which is what makes you jumpy and on-edge. Constantly trying to shut that down could lead to feeling emotionally cold and removed.

There are medications that can help you stop thinking about and reacting to what happened, including the occurrence of nightmares and flashbacks. However, often there are side effects that may make your condition even worse. Be thorough when considering this option, and evaluate the risk of side effects versus any potential benefits.

From the National Center for PTSD:

SSRIs (selective serotonin reuptake inhibitors) and SNRIs (serotonin-norepinephrine reuptake inhibitors) are types of antidepressant medication. Medications have two names: a brand name (for example, Zoloft) and a generic name (for example, Sertraline). There are four SSRIs/SNRIs that are recommended for PTSD:

- Sertraline (Zoloft)
- Paroxetine (Paxil)
- Fluoxetine (Prozac)
- Venlafaxine (Effexor)

There are other types of antidepressant medications, but these four medications listed above are the ones that are most effective for PTSD. Much of the above came from the WebMD article linked above. EMDR is from my experiences with it.

Taking only medications without doing therapy can be hurtful rather than helpful. Sadly, many of our veterans are taking unacceptably huge amounts of medications, which in my estimation, makes things worse. It is important not to be over medicated.

Here is some information from a news article done in 2014 by CBS News. "There's an overuse of narcotics," said Dr. Phyllis Hollenbeck, a physician at the VA medical center in Jackson, Mississippi. "It's the first reflex for pain." The people in charge said, 'We want you to sign off on narcotic prescriptions on patients you don't see.' Dr. Hollenbeck said, "I was absolutely stunned. And I knew immediately it was illegal. It works on the surface. It keeps the veterans happy. They don't complain. They're not coming in as often if they have their pain medicine. And the people in charge don't care if it's done right."

CBS News obtained VA data through a records request which showed the number of prescriptions written by VA doctors and nurse practitioners during the past eleven years. The number of patients treated by VA is up twenty nine percent, but narcotics prescriptions are up 259 percent.

A dozen VA physicians who've worked at fifteen VA medical centers told us they've felt pressured by administrators to prescribe narcotics and that patients are not being properly monitored.

"I have seen people that have not had an exam of that body part that they're complaining of pain in for two years," said a doctor who presently treats pain patients at the VA and asked not to be identified.

"It's easier to write a prescription for narcotics, and just move along, get to the next patient."

"We're letting people come in and prescribing massive doses of narcotics and they also are on drugs for mental health problems," the doctor continued.

By giving those kinds of quantities of pills, one might assume that requires a rather close eye to be kept on the patient. "You would think so. But it isn't the case," said the doctor. From https://www.cbsnews.com/news/veterans-dying-from-overmedication/

Here is a link to another report on VA care and medications: https://www.youtube.com/watch?v=6DmZqVluIxE

A federal investigation confirmed what CBS News reported on last year: that many wounded veterans are being overmedicated in VA hospitals. Some overdoses have been fatal. The Inspector General in the Department of Veterans Affairs discovered the problem is widespread.

The VA's Inspector General found:

- Ninety three percent of long-term narcotics patients were also on a sedative called benzodiazepine. When mixed, the two drugs put patients at an increased risk of fatal overdose.
- Only nine percent of VA patients taking narcotics were seen by a pain clinic.
- Less than half of narcotics patients on multiple drugs had their medications reviewed by VA staff.

Since CBS News broke the story, the VA says it has initiated some reforms and 40,000 fewer veterans are now being prescribed narcotics. The department also says more comprehensive pain management approaches are being implemented at VA hospitals around the country. From: https://www.cbsnews.com/news/vas-overmedication-of-vets-widespread-inspector-general-finds/

VA hospitals have been given the nickname "candyland" because of all the narcotics they prescribe for veterans. In August of 2014, Jason Simcakoski, a former Corporal in the Marines, died as a result of a cocktail of thirteen + medications all prescribed by the VA.

In 2016, DisabledVeterans.org stated, according to a study, that "Veterans receiving polypharmacy (five or more psychotropic drugs administered concurrently) treatments may be at the center of the mystery. Those veterans who receive polypharmacy treatments were four times more likely to commit suicide." Another study showed that veterans who seek mental health care through the VA are MORE likely to kill themselves than those who do not.
https://www.disabledveterans.org/2016/11/07/criminal-overmedication-veterans-causing-suicides/

There is a genetic test that can stop this— over and mixed medication epidemic in its tracks. The VA has already approved this type of drug sensitivity test and they are even currently using it, but just not applying it to the veteran's medication process. The <u>veteran must ask for the test</u> either through their VA doctor or contact any contracted company to receive the test. As a caveat, these companies with VA contracts have stipulations that don't allow them to advertise their presence in the VA. Without tests like these, doctors can only prescribe using methods dictated by bureaucrats and Big Pharma oversight. If a veteran is on two or more medications daily, or on an opioid, blood thinner, or psychotropic drug; they should be required by the VA to take a drug sensitivity test. These tests save medication expense and could save veterans lives. From:
https://sofrep.com/news/va-overmedicating-veterans/

I do not see that veterans truly have access to this sensitivity test.

Bottom line is that unless you need medication to do the therapy to heal your trauma, it is safer not to use it. If you are going to use medication, please be monitored by a physician or prescribing nurse psychotherapist and do review all the side effects before you decide to use a medication. Sometimes the effects and side effects of medication are worse than the symptoms of the PTSD. If you are taking more than one medication, find out how the different medications interact with each other before you take them.

We have already talked about how attitudes and beliefs effect your success and here are some more things to consider. In the prologue to his book, *The Biology of Belief,* Bruce Lipton Ph.D., states: "I was exhilarated by the new realization that I could change the character of my life by changing my beliefs…I realized that there was a science-based path that would take me from my job as a perennial 'victim' to my new job as 'cocreator' of my destiny." He says in the book that fear shuts down a person's growth, and the opposite, love, promotes growth. In addition, he goes into depth about the newly discovered fact that genes do NOT determine our destiny — our environment and beliefs do. All that is to say, YOU are in charge of your life and the outcomes of your choices and actions.

Dr. Lipton goes further and identifies energy fields that impact our physiology and health and how those fields impact biological regulation. He goes into depth about the positive and negative effects of medications and the differences between Newtonian and Quantum mechanics. In his book, *Biology of Belief,* Dr. Lipton explores the differences between our conscious and subconscious mind and which has greater power over us. He describes how we can change our unhealthy programming.

While his book is primarily about cell biology, there is so much more in it. He explores beliefs and their effects on our biology, even in regard to the use of medications. "When we change our beliefs, we change the blood's neurochemical composition, which initiates a complementary change in the body's cells." He cites a study that measured the effects of Mindfulness in changing vital gene functions. He also describes the fight/flight function in us and how it affects our life sustaining energy, our immune system and our ability to think clearly. Dr. Lipton revealed new research that shows successful recovery from PTSD is highly associated with perceived social support.

Our memories are not only in our mind but also in our cells. To heal the traumatic experiences that often lead to PTSD, we need to clear them from both our mind and our cells. Energy psychology/Energy physiology can show the way for that. Both EMDR and EFT fit into that category of energy psychology.

It is my hope that my story and this book has served you and will help you understand PTSD, its impact on your body, mind, and life, but most importantly, how to heal from it. Imagine how your life will be enhanced when you are healed.

# REFERENCES

https://www.ptsd.va.gov/understand/what/ptsd_basics.asp
https://www.ptsd.va.gov/professional/treat/essentials/dsm5_ptsd.asp
https://www.ptsd.va.gov/professional/treat/essentials/history_ptsd.asp
https://www.nimh.nih.gov/health/topics/post-traumatic-stress-disorder-ptsd/index.shtml

*The Biology of Belief*, Bruce Lipton, PH.D. Hay House, 2005
*The Body Keeps the Score*, Bessel Van Der Kolk. Penguin Books 2014
*Trauma and Recovery*, Judith Herman, M.D., Basic Books, 1997

# APPENDIX

## GROUP THERAPY CONTRACT

I, _____ am making the following agreements with the intention of keeping them. I understand that I will not be perfect and that I am responsible for being accountable to my group and therapists. When I break these agreements, I also understand that if I intentionally and /or repeatedly break these agreements, especially in a serious or dangerous way, or, if I refuse to be accountable for a broken agreement, I may be asked to leave the group.

I. SELF-CARE CONTRACTS

    A. I will not harm myself, others, or my environment, nor provoke or allow others to harm me accidentally or on purpose no matter what. I WILL BE SAFE AND HONOR THE SAFETY OF OTHERS AND MY ENVIRONMENT.

    B. I will not run away physically or emotionally, I WILL STAY IN THERAPY, BE FULLY PRESENT, AND WORK THROUGH AND SOLVE MY PROBLEMS.

    C. I will not get sick or go crazy. I WILL BE SANE AND HEALTHY.

    D. I will not be sneaky or lie. I WILL BE HONEST WITH MYSELF AND OTHERS BOTH EMOTIONALLY AND INTELLECTUALLY.

    E. I will not be passive. I WILL BE RESPONSIVE AT ALL TIMES AND I WILL CONFRONT PASSIVITY IN OTHERS AND ACCEPT CONFRONTATION FROM OTHERS.

    F. I am accountable for my feelings, thoughts and actions. I understand that if I break any of these self-care contracts, I will be accountable to myself and my group members. I will use the accountability structure and review my thinking with a minimum of two group members.

## II. GROUP ATTENDANCE

A. I understand that for my therapy to be successful, I must make it my top priority. Therefore, I will be on time and attend every group. The only exceptions are:

1. Scheduled vacations that I write on the "miss list." Spontaneous Vacations are supported when they are a healthy self-care measure and checked out in advance of the missed session.
2. Contagious illness.
3. Death or serious illness of someone close to me.
4. Valid other reason I check out in advance with therapist, e.g. a. An occasional required work absence. b. A serious emergency (emergency defined jointly with therapist)

**MISSED GROUPS WITH NO NOTICE MAY BE CONSIDERED RUNNING!**

B. In case of a planned absence of any kind, I will arrange in advance to attend an alternate group when possible to get support.
C. If I miss group, I am responsible for contacting group members to get any pertinent information (dates, contracts, changes, etc.) given during the missed session, prior to attending the next group.
D. I will not attend group after consuming mind-altering substances.

## III. INDIVIDUAL RESPONSIBILITY

A. I accept ultimate responsibility for the progress and results of my therapy. I will ask for and get the support and guidance I need from my therapists and group. I understand the philosophy that the more I invest in my group process the more I will benefit.
B. I accept complete and full responsibility for my own personal safety on the property located at

_____. I also agree to be responsible for any damage I may cause there.

C. I understand that when I choose to participate in bodywork, there is strenuous physical activity and risk involved. I will accept coaching and protection from the therapists and myself and act responsibly. I agree to use and honor the "1,2,3, Stop" signal.

D. I have been informed that touch is an important part of this therapy and it is intended to be therapeutic and protective. At **no time will this touching be abusive or sexual in nature.** I understand and accept that **I retain the ultimate power and responsibility for when and how I am touched and by whom.**

E. Prior to joining group, I will inform the therapists of any and all known personal addictions or addictive behavior. If I am recovering, I will be clear and share with the group how I am maintaining my sobriety/abstinence, etc. I understand that sobriety is essential to my ability to utilize this process.

F. I will inform the therapists and group members of any communicable illness that I have and I will be ethical and considerate in my contact with others.

G. I understand that as I make personal changes the dynamics in many of my relationships will also change. I will get the support and information I need from my therapists to stay clear with the important people in my life.

H. I will pay each month for group unless I have made other arrangements. Any balance not paid within ninety days will automatically be sent through a computerized collection system.

## IV. GROUP RULES

A. **I will honor the privacy and confidentiality of the therapists and group members** by not revealing anything that takes place in group, that could in any way identify a person or their therapeutic process. When talking with group members away from the group room, I will not name anyone from group. I know that I may talk about myself, my own experiences in group, but not talk about others or their work in any way which identifies them. I may share announcements with group members who missed group. If I choose to share my own process with someone outside of group, I am advised that by so doing, <u>I may risk being misunderstood by someone who does not have sufficient information and experiential context for my work. This is brought to my attention not to promote secrecy, but rather to protect me while I am in therapy, so that my group is a safe place for me and communication in group is enhanced</u>.

B. **I will not be violent in any way to a person or thing except in the context of a contract to do so.** I will arrange for the safe expression of my feelings. I will accept responsibility for any damage I cause. I will honor, at all times, without exception, the established signal for immediate termination of any procedure.

V. TERMINATION

A. Before terminating for any reason, I will give at least three weeks' notice, and follow the accepted "check out" process. The ways of terminating are:

> Leave of Absence – when it is appropriate for logistical, personal or psychotherapeutic reasons for me to suspend my active participation in group therapy for a defined period.

1. Graduation – when, to the best of my current knowledge, I have completed my therapy in this form.

B. If I miss group for more than two weeks, without prior agreement, it will be assumed that I am "running" and I will forfeit my place in group. I understand that I am responsible for paying for those two weeks.

C. If I miss **three** consecutive weeks without prior agreement, I understand that my **participation in group is automatically terminated and the door closes behind me so that I may not return.**

**I HAVE READ THE PRECEDING CONTRACT AND I UNDERSTAND THAT MY RESPONSIBILITY IS TO KEEP ALL OF THESE AGREEMENTS TO THE VERY BEST OF MY ABILITY. I AGREE TO ACKNOWLEDGE, DEAL WITH AND LEARN FROM MY MISTAKES WHILE I AM IN THIS PROCESS.**

_____

SIGNED                                    DATE

_____

THERAPIST                                 DATE

## **THINK STRUCTURE**

(1) I am feeling _____
                (Mad, Scared, Sad, Glad)

(2) Because I think if I _____
                (Behavior I initiate)

(3) I will be _____
                (Negative response)

(4) Instead of _____
                (Positive response)

(5) So I _____
                (Adaptive behavior)

## **AFFIRMATION**

(1) I do _____

(2) And I am _____

## PHANTASY CHECK OUT

May I check out a phantasy with you?
My phantasy is that you do not like me. Is there any truth to that?
My phantasy is that when you told me you had other plans for Saturday night that you were not being totally truthful and that you did not want to spend time with me. Is there any truth to that?

## YOUR RIGHTS AS A CLIENT

As a member of this group, I have the following rights:

1. To be treated in a manner that promotes dignity and self-respect.

2. To be treated without discrimination regarding race color, age, national origin, religion, gender or sexual preference.

3. To be treated without discrimination for mental or physical disability unless such disability makes participation in the group disadvantageous or detrimental to me.

4. To have all information treated confidentially.

## CLEARING STRUCTURE

From time to time, you may find that you need to speak up and be an advocate for yourself or your inner child, or clear something between you and another person so that you can be close. These are times to do a clearing. The structure to use is as follows:

I FEEL _____

(Mad, Sad, Scared)

BECAUSE I BELIEVE THAT WHEN

_____

(Behavior, Experience)

THAT MEANS TO ME

_____

(About me/phantasy)

WHAT I NEED FROM YOU

_____

WHAT I NEED FROM MYSELF

_____

Clearings can also be misused.
In order to be sure you don't misuse it, check in with yourself before doing a clearing by asking these questions:

1. Am I acting as if I am more important than others?
2. Has my nurturing and structuring parent abandoned my kid?
3. Am I operating out of the old belief structure rather than the new one?
4. Am I trying to shift responsibility for action to someone else rather than using the knowledge and skills I have?

5. Am I into a "gotcha" game?
6. Have I been inconsiderate?
7. Am I too unclear to clear?
8. Is the amount of energy I am feeling out of proportion to what I am wanting to clear about?
9. Am I trying to force my beliefs about how to be in the world onto the other person rather than respecting their lifestyle?
10. Have I set this situation up?
11. Am I doing this to provoke or test the other person?
12. Can I do this clearing outside of group?
13. Am I sabotaging or avoiding my work by spending my time clearing?
14. Is this clearing for some purpose other than helping me be fully present?

**IF YOU ANSWERED YES TO ANY OF THESE – DON'T DO A CLEARING!**

## TYPES OF WORK

Trust fall
Trust lift
"No" saying
Energy Moving
Energy Releasing
Body work
Boundary Work
Breathwork
Break In
Gestalt work
Psychodrama
Trance work
Anger Work
Towel Pull
Sheet Pull
Pushing
Pounding
Tearing
Clay work
Guided Imagery

These were discovered and developed in process by both clients and therapists. This is not an exhaustive list. Be creative and discover what you need and ask for help to manifest how it can work. You are not limited.

# EFT
## EMOTIONAL FREEDOM TECHNIQUE

The brain and body do not know the difference between past and present. All the wartime memories, including sense stimuli, live in the cells of the body. Anything can trigger the release of the memories with full intensity. Those triggers are unpredictable and catch the veteran off guard. Once triggered, they/you can relive the trauma as though it is currently happening. They/you are no longer in current physical reality. Trauma leads to the need to control the environment, yet when there are many unpredictable triggers, it adds to the stress and distress the veteran experiences. When the limbic system is constantly overwhelmed, the veteran does not have access to their ability to think, problem-solve and act rationally.

EFT neutralizes the chemical and physiological reactions in the body to traumatic memories and pain. Trauma and anxiety disrupt the flow of energy through the body and EFT restores the balance. EFT can also reprogram the subconscious beliefs.

EFT can rewire the disturbing memories that recur from trauma and break the connection between the memories and body reactions. Symptoms are caused by a disruption in the energy system and EFT restores balance. EFT can reduce symptoms of anxiety, depression, panic, insomnia, headaches, and feeling out of control. It creates a feeling of calm and restores more normal functioning.

1. When triggered, begin by identifying how intense the symptoms are on a scale of 0 -10. 0=none and 10=highest level.
2. Tap the points listed while saying what you are thinking and feeling. Keep tapping and moving to the next point.
3. You may also state, "Even though I have this (any symptoms, or issue) I can get through this and feel and function better or I know I am OK and will remain OK. I deeply and completely love and accept myself."

4. Male veterans may resist the last statement but are encouraged to work with it nonetheless. The statement by itself, using the points, is healing and reprograms the subconscious negative self-beliefs.
5. POINTS
    a. KC - Karate Chop – side of hand between wrist and bottom of little finger.
    b. EB - Eyebrow – inner corner of both eyebrows.
    c. SE - Side of Eye – outside groove over bone. Both sides.
    d. UE - Under the eye at 45° angle in middle of bone. Both.
    e. UN - Under the nose and between upper lip and nose.
    f. CH - Chin between the lower lip and chin.
    g. CB - Collar Bone – Just under the two collarbones slide fingers on diagonal to find little divots or use flat part of fingers with fist over sternum between collarbones.
    h. UA - Under your arm about where the seam of your shirt is and between your waist and the middle of under your arm. Use all fingers.
    i. TH - Top of your head slightly back of middle. Use all fingers.

After one round, measure intensity again and keep going until the intensity is at 0. After one or more rounds if you wish you may change the statement to: "Even though I <u>still have some</u> (issues or symptoms) I know it is not necessary and I deserve to feel better. I deeply and completely love and accept myself."

**Phrases to use:**
"Even though I (killed those …..) and was ordered to do so, I violated my own values and have felt the guilt from that. I now release it. I have punished myself enough. I deeply and completely love and accept myself."

"Even though I could not save (Red's life/…….) and feel guilty, I am not responsible for the outcome — only my own intention and behavior. I choose to let go of the guilt and the pain I have carried. I deeply and completely love and accept myself."

"Even though I could not stop the rapist or the rape, I know it is not my fault and I can now live and live fully. I deeply and completely love and accept myself."

"Even though I participated in that horrific (traumatic, inappropriate, violent, ...) event/experience I can now forgive my younger self for that, and my older self for judging and criticizing myself. I choose life and deeply and completely love and accept myself."

## SOME LETTERS I WROTE HOME on the following pages

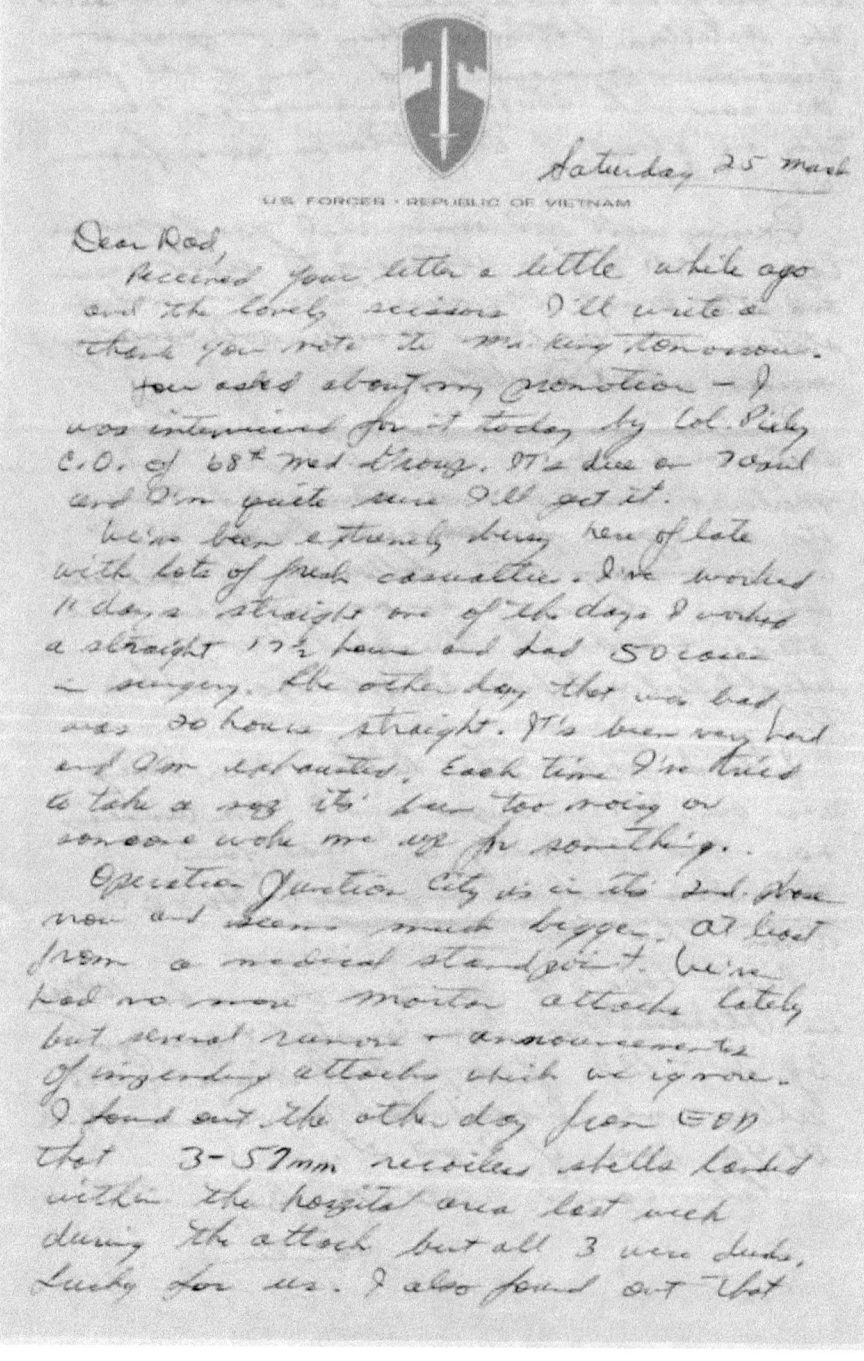

the surgeons complained to our C.O. about the artillery bothering them in surgery, so division command had them moved from across the street permanently. Now they are about 4 city blocks away from us.

Bunny sent me some real good music tapes which I am listening to right now and it's great because the one radio station we have plays mostly roll & country music which I detest.

I was supposed to go to Chu Loi last week for a party but due to the mortar attack it was cancelled. Now it's on again for next friday & it's a swimming party followed by cocktails, dinner & dancing & an overnight pass with steak & eggs for breakfast. It sounds delightful & I hope it goes through this time.

I heard about the Riots you having over our news report and I am wondering how bad it really is? Was your store damaged in any way? How is it down there now?

I am hoping to go to a luau on 10 May in Pleiku. I've been invited & can go by C-130 if my chief nurse will allow me. I need her permission. I'll let you know if I get it.

Take care. All my love
Saralee

18 April 67

1st CAVALRY DIVISION
U.S. Armed Forces - Vietnam

Dear Dad,

Received watch OK, still have it. Had a chance to see the girl yet to show it to her. I decided if she doesn't want it someone else may. Thank you for sending it. I'll let you know as soon as I sell it.

What do you mean the Miami Herald is doing a story on me? Why? What have I done. The ad you had put in the Ft. Lauderdale news I really didn't care for too much because I don't think it's a good idea to publish my location and also the news of the mortar attack & the shells landing in the hospital area might frighten someone or if they knew anyone at the 12th Evac. What if some big Army cheese sees it? I might get into trouble for writing that to you. I hope no trouble comes from it. I have received 3 letters in response to the ad and I must admit all very nice. One was from Mrs. Florida 1961 Monelle Matthews, 1011 N.E.

27th Terrace, Pompano Beach. She wrote a very nice letter commending our youth that serve and said that the riot news was exaggerated. The best letter though was from a Mr. John O. Leonard of 910 N.E. 17th Way #8, Ft. Lauderdale, Fla. He said he didn't know about the trouble till he heard it on the news. He said Dade County news radio is prejudiced and reports the news that way because they are jealous of Ft. Lauderdale. He further said that the "local officials" of Ft. Lauderdale could take a few lessons in learning how to handle crowds on the street — he sounded as though he felt some of it could have been provoked by the police. Also he added that many of the "kids" were locals.

He went on to suggest the "kids" spend money & perhaps the city fathers of Ft. Lauderdale could provide an outlet for their energy & perhaps plan ahead for next year. He added that they all looked like good kids who perhaps would be in Viet Nam before to long and would probably make a good showing.

The last part of his letter was the

**1st CAVALRY DIVISION**
*U.S. Armed Forces Vietnam*

Dear,

"You tell all these guys in the hospital that they will get a fair shake when this is all over. We've got the best system in the world — as long as we strive to uphold the rights of the individual, they just can't beat us.

All these draft dodgers, beatniks & Berkeley sit-downers are the "Mothey kids," they'll be lost in the shuffle. You are doing a fine job & we are all proud of you! May the good Lord bless all of you.

It's nice to know there are people back home who stand behind us. We like to feel that there are people who care that we are free to protect our backyards in the U.S.A. It's great to know there are some real Americans back home. It's wonderful to know our young soldiers who give life & limb for their country are appreciated by their fellow countrymen. We come from the greatest country in the world & we want to keep it that way. That's why we're here now.

I did read the letter from
dear Dorothy & I shall write
tonight. I'm sorry that I forgot
to write but I was sure I had
written to her when I first arrived.
Perhaps I'm wrong. I'll try to
do better.

The rains have started here now
& it's an ocean of H2O & a sea of
mud. My roof leaks & my cot
is wet in the O.R. The floors
are flooded & the steril packs
are all wet. We had mass casualties
again today — coming from Duc Hoa
1st 27th infantry. It's very depressing.
This afternoon a Surgeon looked at
me & said — what'll I do as we
looked a a young boy's leg that
was gangrenous & we both knew it
had to come off. The Dr. said — Oh
I want to go home — this poor kid —
and his nurse just cried (me) and
off came the leg and we neither of us
felt very good. Yesterday we fought
to save a young guy whose both
legs were blown off and we failed.
Then a V.C. was brought in & we
saved him — why?  So the
ARVN's can kill him later.

# ABOUT THE AUTHOR

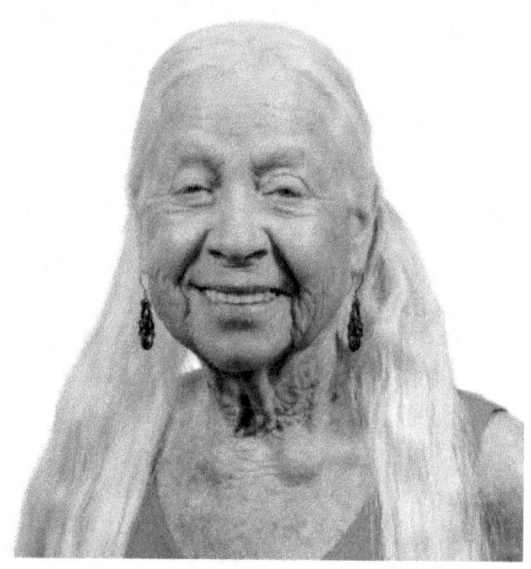

Sarah L. Blum is a decorated nurse Vietnam veteran who earned the Army Commendation Medal serving as an operating room nurse during the height of the fighting in 1967. She received her Bachelor's Degree from Seattle University and her Master's from U. W. At age 80, Sarah retired after more than 34 years healing trauma. Between 2006 and 2012, Sarah interviewed over 58 women veterans and is the author of *Women Under Fire: Abuse in the Military* about the culture of abuse toward women in the U.S. Military. *Warrior Nurse, Healer: PTSD and Healing* is her second book. Sarah has a third degree black belt in Aikido, was a rower and coxswain for a rowing club, and loves playing African drums.

# NOTE FROM SARAH L. BLUM

Word-of-mouth is crucial for any author to succeed. If you enjoyed *Warrior Nurse*, please leave a review online—anywhere you are able. Even if it's just a sentence or two. It would make all the difference and would be very much appreciated.

Thanks!
Sarah L. Blum

We hope you enjoyed reading this title from:

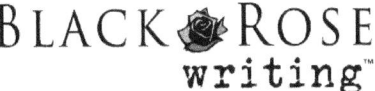

www.blackrosewriting.com

Subscribe to our mailing list – *The Rosevine* – and receive **FREE** books, daily deals, and stay current with news about upcoming releases and our hottest authors.
Scan the QR code below to sign up.

Already a subscriber? Please accept a sincere thank you for being a fan of Black Rose Writing authors.

View other Black Rose Writing titles at www.blackrosewriting.com/books and use promo code **PRINT** to receive a **20% discount** when purchasing.